# Disorders of Voice

MARGARET C. L. GREENE

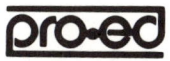

5341 Industrial Oaks Boulevard
Austin, Texas 78735

**The PRO-ED
studies in
communicative disorders**

*Series editor*
HARVEY HALPERN

Copyright © 1986 by PRO-ED, Inc.
Printed in the United States of America.
All rights reserved. No part of this book may be reproduced in any form or by any means without the prior written permission of the publisher.

**Library of Congress Cataloging in Publication Data**
Greene, Margaret C. L.
  Disorders of voice.

  (The Pro-Ed studies in communicative disorders)
  Rev. ed. of: The voice and its disorders. 4th ed. 1980.
  Bibliography: p.
  1. Voice disorders. 2. Voice  I. Greene, Margaret C. L. Voice and its disorders. II. Title. III. Series.
  RF510.G73    1986    616.85'5    86-489
  ISBN 0-89079-092-2

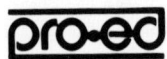

5341 Industrial Oaks Boulevard
Austin, Texas 78735

10 9 8 7 6 5 4 3 2 1          86 87 88 89 90 91

# Contents

Preface ... v

## PART ONE
Normal Voice ... 1

Aspects of Voice ... 2
Characteristics of Normal Voice ... 4
Anatomy and Physiology of Voice Production ... 4

## PART TWO
Dysphonia ... 15

Assessment ... 15
Instruments in Vocal Assessment ... 16
Classification of Voice Disorders ... 18
Management of Hyperkinetic Dysphonia ... 24
Rehabilitation for Hyperkinetic Dysphonia ... 27
Psychological (Functional) Dysphonia ... 31
Systemic Disorders ... 35
Endocrine Disorders ... 38
Structural Anomalies and Abnormalities ... 41
Neurological Disorders ... 43
Tumors of the Larynx ... 49
Laryngectomy and Esophageal Speech ... 50
Surgical Speech Restoration ( Fistula Voice) ... 54
References ... 59

# Preface

This monograph is devised as an introduction to the serious problems which affect communication when there is a breakdown in normal voice production. The attributes of normal voice and their importance in speech are described, and the theme "the voice is the person" is emphasized. A simple account with diagrams is provided of the anatomy and physiology of the vocal instrument and how phonation produced in the larynx is embellished by inflection, rhythm, volume, and resonance. The reader is then introduced to a series of voice disorders commonly encountered by speech pathologists—explaining in simple terms the etiology, phonatory symptoms, and suggestions for rehabilitation.

*Disorders of Voice* will prove a valuable introduction to dysphonia for student speech pathologists who can follow up the extensive references provided for study in depth. It is also intended that the text will be a reliable guide to doctors, nurses, social workers, teachers, and all those who require further information on the management of dysphonia.

# PART ONE

## Normal Voice

In order to appreciate the importance of voice in speech, it is helpful to contemplate what it is like to be without a voice—being only able to whisper. One of the primary functions of voice is to make speech audible to an audience and against background noise. At some time in their lives, most individuals have experienced total loss of voice (aphonia) and severe hoarseness (dysphonia) when suffering from a bad cold and laryngitis. The feelings of frustration, helplessness, embarrassment, and irritation at not being heard and understood remain a vivid and unpleasant memory long after return to vocal health. Being unable to laugh, for example, is traumatic.

The voice, however, has many other important assets besides that of volume. The voice conveys meaning since it plays a role in the linguistic aspects of speech, marking stress and intonation patterns. Being a musical instrument, the voice has aesthetic and artistic features and, being as characteristic of an individual as that individual's face and person, it is a part of the personality and tied to the emotional and psychological development of a human being. The voice is, in a very real way, the person you are as well as the person you meet and know.

The voice provides a musical accompaniment to speech, and its rhythm, stress, volume changes, length of phrase, and speed of delivery are distinctive features of effective and clear discourse. These features are distinct from the phonetic features of pronunciation of vowels and consonants in words (articulatory aspects) and the grammatical, syntactic, and semantic features (linguistic aspects). The linguistic message can in fact be executed in a featureless and monotonous drone lacking life and impact, but its meaning will not be very clear.

# Aspects of Voice

## Pitch

A very obvious feature of voice is its pitch, which throughout life matches sex and age. The childish trebles of boys and girls are similar, but during puberty, with increase in body size and development of sexual characteristics, boys develop male voices and girls female ones. As years go by, the voice matures and its quality changes naturally as the muscles age and their resilience and contour change—a process that we recognize and accept (Greene, 1982; Mysak & Hanley, 1959; Oyer & Oyer, 1976). A high pitch in a mature male and a girlish voice in a woman indicate immaturity and some problem in personality structure.

## Rhythm

Rhythm (stress) is so important in speech that, when it is lost, speech becomes incomprehensible, as in the extreme example of festinating speech in individuals with Parkinson's disease. The rapid speech of the clutterer (Weiss, 1960) can also be difficult to understand. Unusual rhythms can render dialects difficult to follow: to an English Southerner, "broad" Glaswegian, Geordie, or Scots can be incomprehensible.

Stress affects the meaning of not only whole but many single words as well (e.g., *entrance, desert, contract, incense*). Many nouns are changed to verbs by the subtle emphasis on the indefinite article (e.g., *a mass, amass; a tune, attune; a bridge, abridge,* and many more).

## Intonation

Stress, melody, and intonation (inflection) are inescapably linked within languages. Intonation is learned very early by the infant and precedes words and phrases; it can be heard in the conversational jargon, the "talking scribble," of the 18-month-old toddler. The flow of syllables reflects the inflections of adult speech and, if not learned very early in life, is never fully mastered. This is why speakers of a foreign language are detected immediately to be foreigners by the natives of a country, despite a perfect command of vocabulary and syntax. The inflections of one's mother tongue are retained in another language. Thus, Indians speaking English with Hindi or Hindustani inflection may be, and often are, incomprehensible to the English as the influence of British Raj "pukka" English grows ever more distant to Indian ears.

## Tone

Intonation and tone of voice are additional important features of verbal communication. A message is often far more significant in how we say it than in what we say. Consider the phrase "Fetch me that book, will you?" This can be uttered with a whole range of meanings—coaxing, exasperation, aggression, bullying, or simply a request envisaging nothing but cooperation. It depends upon the relationship existing at the moment between the two personalities involved, as well as the situation and the role of each person within it: teacher and child, child and friend, librarian and assistant, parent and child, and so on. The voice reflects feelings based on primitive, deep layers of personality and reactions to others. These feelings often give us away since they are so hard to conceal.

## Quality

Each voice is as singular to the speaker as the face. It is comparable to the fingerprint, since it bears the stamp of an individual's anatomy. The structural characteristics of the vocal tract shape the qualities of voice while personality and emotional reactions mold these qualities still further. Actors who are truly successful, although unable to change the anatomical quality of their voices, can change their emotional expression, actually impersonating the role of Hamlet or Macbeth. But the voice of an Olivier or Gielgud, though changed, is instantly recognizable, just as these actors may assume appropriate facial expressions but their faces remain their own.

The natural voice of an individual thus tells us much about the personality besides identifying who is speaking. A strong voice, clear and purposeful, reflects a person who has self-confidence and high self-esteem. A mumbling, quiet, or breathy voice reflects feelings of inferiority and a desire for self-effacement. Restless, rapid speech with exaggerated inflections and brittle tone probably denotes anxiety, just as a slow, monotonous delivery may be due to extreme fatigue or deep depression (Moses, 1954).

The average person probably takes note of the voices of individuals largely unconsciously, but the undertones of speech must contribute to an evaluation of a new acquaintance and thus may account for many of our immediate likes and dislikes, a factor a speech pathologist must recognize in contact with clients. The extraordinary intuition displayed by some people is undoubtedly connected with their having good ears for reading the subliminal score. Though it comes naturally to some, it can be acquired through experience and is essential in the art of speech therapy and vocal rehabilitation.

## Characteristics of Normal Voice

A normal voice is hard to define. It has to be audible, pleasant in tone, not too loud or too soft, and appropriate to the sex, age, and socioeconomic background of the individual. But for all these features there are flexible boundaries for what is normal and acceptable, largely dictated by circumstances and environment. A television or radio news announcer, a preacher, or a teacher should not have a harsh or hoarse voice, but this may be entirely acceptable in an auctioneer, a bookie, or a market stall vendor. In some environments a cultivated voice may give offense as an affectation, placing the speaker and listener in different social classes. Subtle indefinable standards of voice reign in different social strata.

An abnormal voice has to be recognized as strange and out of the ordinary by everybody concerned, regardless of race, rank, or education. Although there are sophisticated electronic machines nowadays capable of individual scientific measurements of pitch, volume, duration, and harmonic structure, there is still no machine that can condense these into a whole—a human voice that fuses anatomic, physiologic, and acoustic properties and personal traits and emotions. Machines have concrete value in scientific measurement but a limited value in assessment and teaching, for they cannot replace the listening ear of an experienced speech therapist. Such qualities as breathiness, hoarseness, strain, harshness, fry, and so on cannot be defined by electronic analysis or verbal description; they remain the subjective judgment of the listener.

## Anatomy and Physiology of Voice Production

Knowledge of the anatomic structures involved in voice production—how the human body works in producing phonation—is vital to the understanding of normal and abnormal function. The voice is produced by a musical wind instrument that functions like any other musical instrument—as a whole, with each activity related to the others. Energy for the sound waves comes from breath from the lungs activating the vocal cords (the vibrator or reed) and producing the fundamental note of a certain pitch and volume. This fundamental note is then

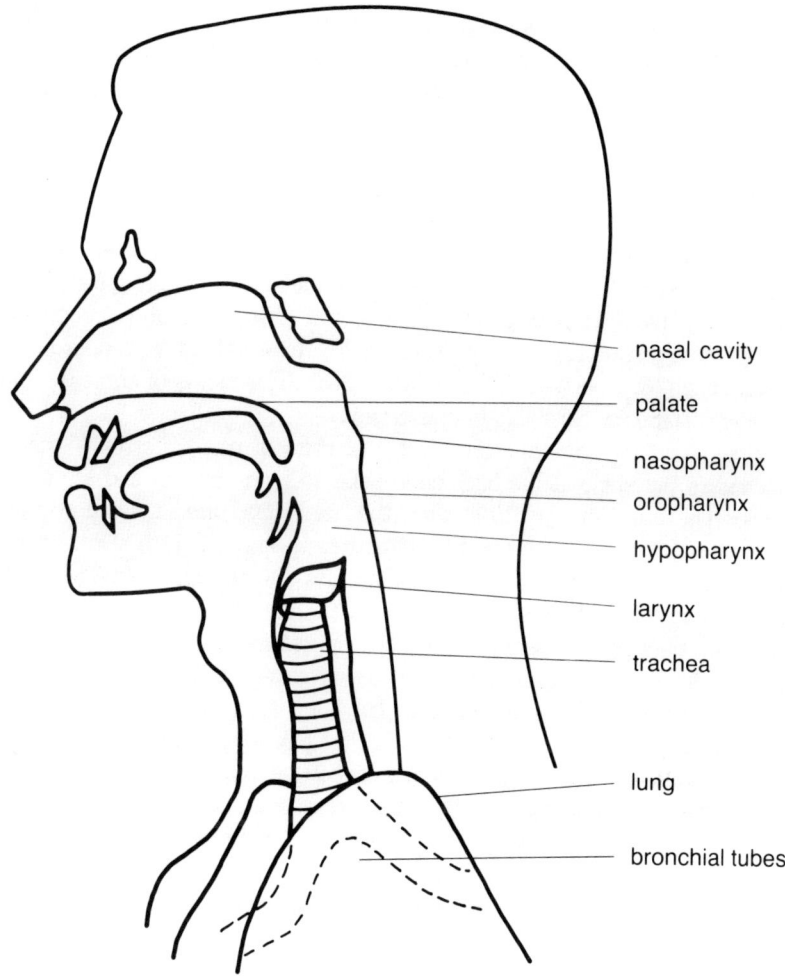

**Figure 1.** The vocal instrument.

resonated and amplified by the flexible walls and air-filled cavities of the chest, neck, and head (see Figure 1).

## The Chest and Lungs

Respiration is vital to life. The human being can survive some 8 weeks without food, 7 days without water, but only 4 minutes without air without incurring suffocation and brain damage. Oxygenation of the blood and expiration of the waste product carbon dioxide takes place through the diffusion of gases in the alveoli of the lungs. Normal breathing patterns are essential to good health, and the importance of breathing control has been recognized in the Eastern philosophies for centuries and in the teaching of relaxation and meditation.

The lungs are emptied and filled by the downward and upward movements of the diaphragm, acting exactly like the diaphragm of a bellows. The diaphragm is actually a passive muscle controlled by the abdominal and intercostal muscles. The outward and inward movements of the chest and the upper abdomen can be felt and consciously controlled in the production of voice and song (Campbell, Agostini, & Newsom-Davis, 1970; Hixon, Mead, & Goldman, 1976; Mead, Hixon, & Goldman, 1974; Wilder, 1983). This fact is of immense importance in respiratory rehabilitation programs.

The chest is a rib cage formed by 12 pairs of ribs. The top 7 pairs are attached to the spine at the back and to the sternum in front and are scarcely mobile. The 8th, 9th, and 10th pairs, the "false ribs," are attached in front to the xiphoid process of the sternum by cartilage, and the 11th and 12th pairs, the "floating ribs," terminate in the abdominal wall (see Figure 2). The contraction of the intercostal muscles that fill the interstices between the ribs elevates them, and they move like bucket handles, increasing the circumference of the thorax. The descent of the diaphragm on inspiration inflates the lungs, which assist in pushing the rib cage outward. The lungs are pear-shaped, larger at the base than at the apexes. These anatomic and physiologic conditions make possible fine control of respiratory volume, air flow, and pressure in the vocal tract in vocalization (Campbell, 1974). The intercostal diaphragmatic method of breathing is generally considered the best for good voice production. Movements of the upper chest need much effort and induce muscular strain due to the enlistment of accessory muscles of the shoulder girdle. This "clavicular breathing" is unavoidable in jogging and other strenuous activities but is harmful if used habitually when at rest, when speaking, and when singing.

In repose, breathing is through the nose, rhythmic and regular. Inspiration and expiration times are equal, with a slight pause at the end of expiration. The average number of respiratory cycles per minute is 12 but may be as low as 8 in repose.

Breathing for speech and song follows another pattern. A quick intake of breath through the mouth, achieved by an accelerated downward pull of the diaphragm that inflates the lungs, precedes speech. Inspiration volume is attuned to the needs of the moment, and expiration time is prolonged according to the length of utterance (i.e., whether a grunt or a rhetorical spate of words).

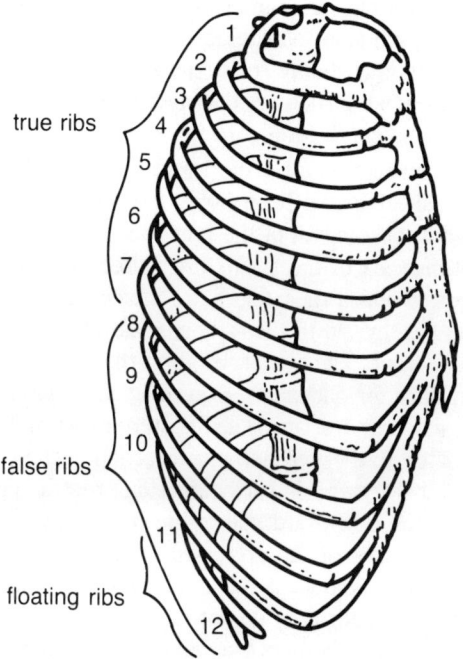

**Figure 2.** The rib cage and thorax.

## The Larynx

The larynx originally developed as a safety valve to close the airway and protect the lungs from entry of saliva and food particles. The epiglottis above channels material to be swallowed down the gullet while the larynx is elevated, and the ventricular folds and vocal cords close firmly to form a watertight seal. Fine control of the muscular vocal cords (the reeds of the vocal wind instrument) through changes of shape, length, and tension produce the changes in pitch and inflections of human speech already described.

The larynx is constructed of cartilages and many highly specialized muscles (see Figures 3 and 4). The base of the larynx is formed by the cricoid cartilage, which is shaped like a signet ring—narrow in front and deep behind—and attached to the top ring of the windpipe. Above the cricoid is suspended the thyroid cartilage, shaped like an open book, with the spine facing forward. This is the Adam's apple; it is larger and more conspicuous in men on account of the larger vocal cords responsible for the deeper voices in males than in females. To the humped back of the cricoid cartilage are attached the triangular-shaped arytenoid cartilages, which are able to slide up and down the cricoid slopes to a limited extent, but more importantly rotate inward and tip forward and backward. The epiglottis is a leaflike structure, the stalk of which is attached to the apex of the posterior cricoid cartilage.

The larynx is suspended from the hyoid bone situated at the root of the tongue; this horseshoe-shaped bone holds the pharyngeal cavity open and is also associated with movements of the tongue in swallowing and speaking.

The internal muscles of the larynx are paired and have names consistent with the cartilages to which their fibers are attached. Thus the thyroarytenoid muscles run from the thyroid to the arytenoid cartilages and span the laryngeal cavity from back to front. These muscles form the vocal cords that are brought together in the midline for phonation. Swivelling and rotating movements of the arytenoids are assisted by the lateral and posterior cricoarytenoid muscles. The arytenoids are shifted to the midline by contraction of the transverse arytenoid muscle. Tilting of the arytenoids backward elongates the cords, an action that can be assisted by the downward pull of the thyroid by the cricothyroid muscles. The vocal processes of the arytenoid cartilages extend one third of the way into the vocal cords, known as the cartilaginous portions. They are approximated for phonation and normally do not take part in the phonatory excursions of the anterior two thirds (the pars vocalis) of the cords but may do so in singing bass notes.

Above the true vocal cords there are small cavities (the laryngeal sinuses) that separate them from the false cords, also known as the vestibular folds but more commonly as the ventricular bands. These bands of muscle are part of the laryngela valvular system and approximate in swallowing; they do not take part in phonation, although they are actually formed by the upper fibers of the thyroarytenoid muscles.

## The Vocals Cords (Folds)

The vocal ligaments are attached to the medial edges of the thyroarytenoids and are white in contrast to the red muscles and the red ventricular bands clearly visible in a laryngoscopic view. The triangular opening in the laryngeal airway formed by the separated vocal cords is known as the glottis—hence the terms *glottal attack* and *glottal stop* used by phoneticians and singers.

The thyroarytenoid muscles forming the bulk of the vocal cords have a very complex structure; their network of fibers running in all directions permits versatile changes in shape. Specialized muscle fibers in the thickened membrane of the vocal ligaments form the vocalis muscles, which are an added means of tensing and relaxing the cords. The bodies of the vocal cords are wedge-shaped,

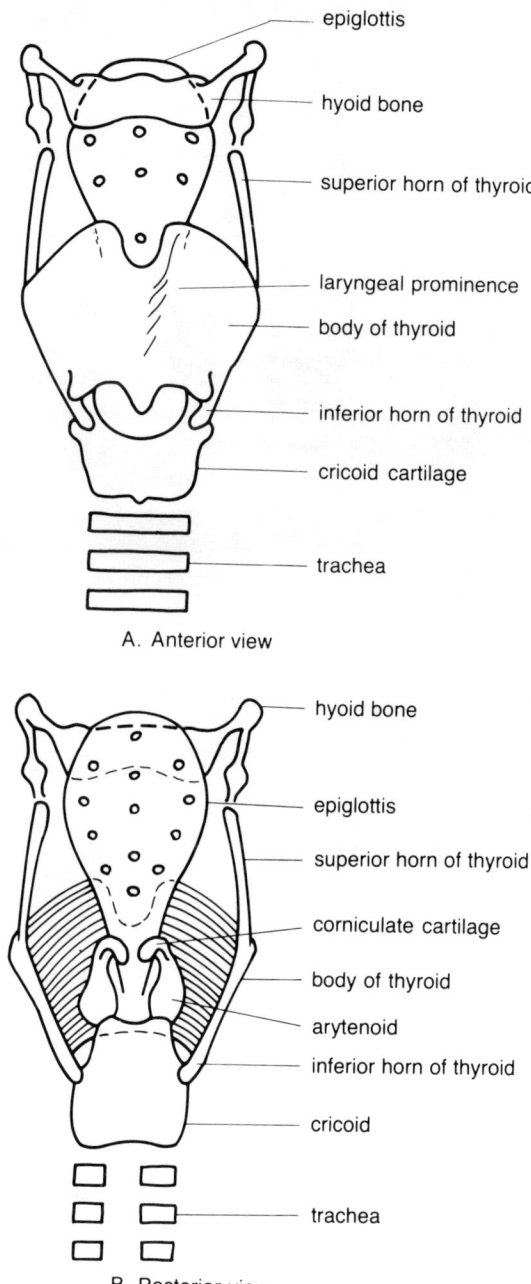

**Figure 3.** Laryngeal structure. A, anterior view; B, posterior view.

10   Disorders of Voice

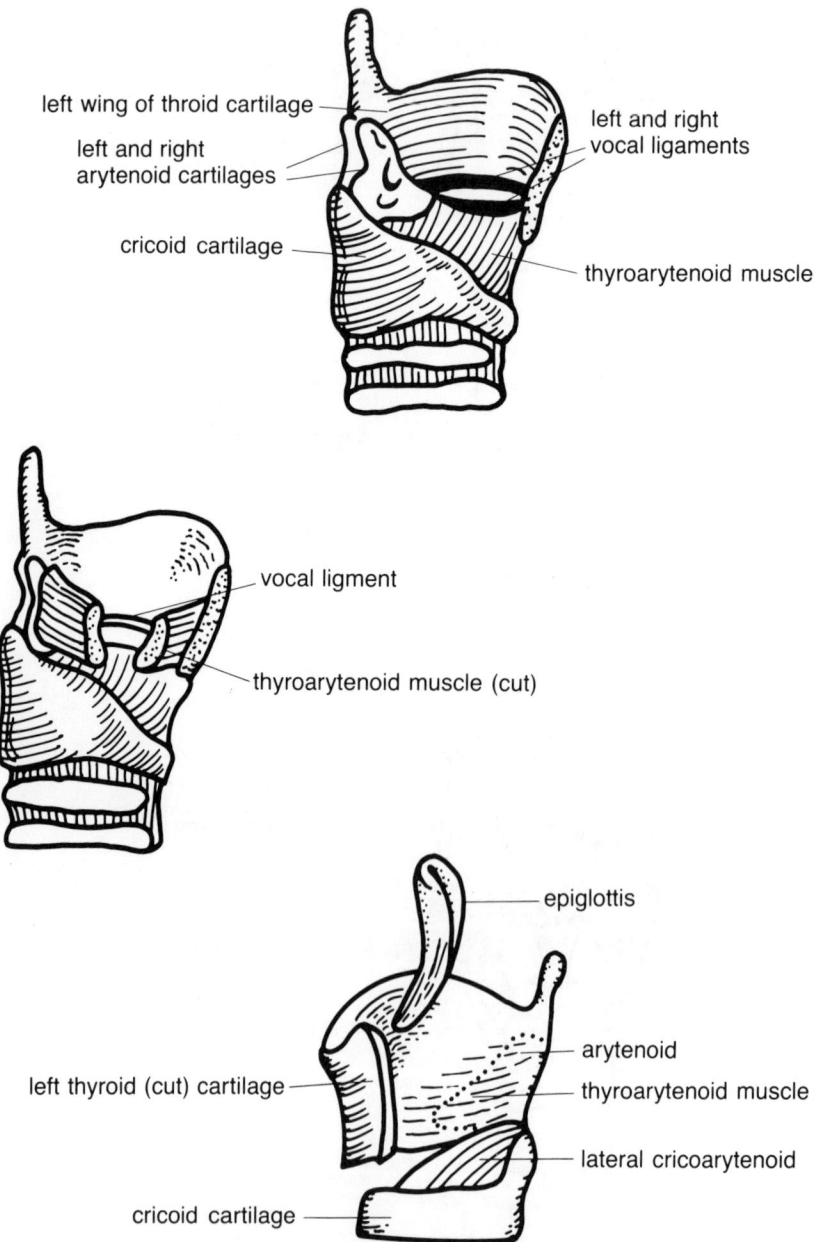

**Figure 4.**   Laryngeal muscles.

but their vibrating edges can become knife-thin for very high notes and present rounded surfaces that roll together on low notes.

The surfaces of the vocal cords are covered by mucous membrane constantly lubricated by mucous glands, which prevents friction between their opposing surfaces in phonation. The vocal folds must just brush each other as they approximate and separate in the vibrating cycles of phonation. The cords are blown apart by the buildup of air pressure beneath them; then they recoil as air escapes in a puff and pressure drops. Each puff of air forms an air wave, a cycle of alternating pressurized and rarefied air particles having properties of size and frequency. Pitch is measured in the number of cycles (or hertz) per second (cps) and volume by decibels—the larger the sound waves, the louder the voice. A note of middle C requires 240 cps. A bass voice has an approximate range of 80–256 cps; a tenor 140–512 cps; and a soprano 384–1,024 cps.

The laryngeal muscles achieve the most delicate adjustments in tension and relaxation with the aid of receptor nerve endings, described by Gould & Okamura (1974) and Wyke (1969; 1974) as spiral in shape encircling individual muscle fibers. Discharges from the nerve endings reflexly facilitate or inhibit muscle tone with great rapidity in different sections of the muscle at the same time (Greene, 1980). Mechanoreceptor reflexes in the laryngeal joints are complementary to the reflex system within the thyroarytenoid muscles, so that exact tuning of the reed vibrator is possible (Bowden, 1974).

## Air Pressure and Air Flow

It is at this point that the relationship between breathing and phonation, between the flow of air from the lungs and pressure below the vocal cords, must be examined (Kelman, Gordon, Simpson, & Morton, 1975).

Large quantities of expired lung air are unnecesary for the production of a loud noise. In fact, extraordinary vocal volume can be produced by extreme muscle tension causing extreme air pressure below the vocal cords as the penetrating yells emanating from the tiny larynges of small infants stand witness (Van den Berg, 1964).

It is not necessary to fill the lungs to capacity, and conversational speech can be produced on residual air after quiet expiration according to Proctor (1972). Singers in times past practiced holding a note so steadily before the flame of a candle that it would not flicker, the unacceptable sign of the escape of unvibrated breath.

Modern technology is able to evaluate more fully the relationship between voice and air flow. Isshiki (1964) studied intensity, subglottic pressure, and air flow. He found that at very low pitch glottal resistance increased with intensity but that flow rate remained fairly constant. On high notes glottal resistance remained almost unchanged while flow rate increased greatly with intensity. Laryngeal control dominated low-pitch intensity, but flow rate controlled by the expiratory muscles dominated high-pitch intensity.

The fact that voice in conversation can be produced by small quantities of air does not mean that in voice training breath training is unimportant. On the contrary. What is crucial is the balance between subglottic pressure and glottic tension. Air flow and buildup of pressure require exact monitoring and control of the respiratory muscles in movements of chest and abdomen. The glottis has to be tuned by ear. Voice production is effortless in normal speakers, but under stress and tension things may go sadly awry in conversational speech. Many professional speakers need training in breath control and voice production if they are to meet the more exacting requirements of lecturing, preaching, acting, singing, or even speaking at length in executive meetings.

## The Resonators

The actual laryngeal note determines the fundamental pitch of the voice, but it is a poor thin sound before it is resonated. The structure of the bodies of all musical instruments determines the characteristic timbre or quality of the musical note it produces. The size and shape, the materials used, and their flexibility all affect the fundamental note produced by the vibrator. The sound is enriched by harmonics, increasing in volume, quality, and carrying power. Notes of the same pitch played on an oboe, flute, or french horn will be quite distinct from each other by reason of the resonance of each instrument. Every resonator responds best to a particular range of notes that it reinforces, while sound waves outside this pitch range are damped and filtered out. The resonator, it is said, "speaks" to notes of optimum pitch. This factor of optimum resonance/pitch is crucial in improving voice production. Power and beauty are added to the voice without extra effort or energy.

The resonators of the voice are all those hollow air-filled cavities above and below the vocal cords. The chest favors the deep notes of male voices and, to a lesser extent, those of contraltos. The vibrations can be felt by placing the fingertips upon the clavicles while a vowel sound is sustained (an important strategy in vocal exercises).

The laryngeal sinuses between the vocal cords and ventricular bands resonate the voice at the outset of its journey up the vocal tract. The larynx then opens into the hypopharynx and the muscular tube of the pharynx proper, which has oral and nasal sections or connections. The nasopharynx is roofed over by the flexible soft palate, which can elevate to meet the posterior pharyngeal wall and prevent the escape of sound waves into the nasal cavity. When there is a palatal-pharyngeal aperture, the voice is nasalized, as in articulation of nasal consonants /m/, /n/, and /ng/.

The soft palate acts as a diaphragm when elevated, however, transmitting sound waves into the nasal cavities and sinuses, which give a brilliance to the voice recognized as head resonance. When this is lacking during a cold or swelling of the nasal mucosa, the voice has a certain dullness. With real nasal obstruction and congestion the nasal consonants are lost and substituted by oral ones, /b/, /d/, and /g/.

The pharyngeal cavity is an all-important resonator, and to be fully effective it should be relaxed and open. Kathleen Ferrier's beautiful voice is said to have been due to her commodious throat, which would accommodate a tennis ball.

The shape and size of the pharynx changes with movements of the back of the tongue that also shift the level of the larynx. The pillars of the fauces are two muscular arches that house the lingual tonsils. Their fibers are inserted into the sides of the tongue and merge with the uvula to form the soft palate. These muscular arches need to be relaxed for successful voice production. Raising the back of the tongue and tensing of the palatal arches give a typical "plummy" quality to speech and shut the voice back in the throat.

The oral cavity is important as a resonator since it is in this region that voice becomes articulate. Movements of the organs of articulation, tongue, teeth, palate, and jaws form consonants, but vowels and diphthongs enhance quality and project the voice (Sundberg, 1970). Mouth shapes and tongue gestures create selective resonators, producing the characteristic resonance frequencies that distinguish vowels and diphthongs from one another. On the other hand, the whole vocal tract from chest to head acts as a "universal resonator."

The oral cavity as a whole resonates and projects the voice forward, acting rather like a megaphone, by increasing volume. As far as is possible, the jaws, lips, and throat should be relaxed and open to allow the free passage of sound waves. Speech experts speak of the need for "open articulation" in speech training, which means chiefly concentration upon vowels and diphthongs. The consonants need fleeting articulatory contacts and direction of sound waves into fricative, sibilant, and plosive sounds.

Finally we must note that although respiration, phonation, and resonation have been described separately, the separate systems are linked and interwoven into a harmonious whole. Being of one piece, the instrument has but one sound, which resonates the personality. The voice is in fact the person.

# PART TWO

# Dysphonia

## Assessment

Dysphonia, a disorder of voice, is recognized as being different from normal voice quite easily by lay people as well as specialists. The etiology of the disorder is not difficult to arrive at with the help of a laryngologist, neurologist, psychiatrist, and speech therapist. What is exceedingly difficult is what appears so easy: the verbal description of the voice and its aberrant qualities. Although Fairbanks (1960) thought the unlimited variety of vocal symptoms presented by patients could be reduced to three categories—harshness, breathiness, and hoarseness—very few experts would agree. Hoarseness may be breathy and harshness may be hoarse; moreover, "harsh" may mean "metallic" (Aronson, 1980). Nasal, rough, gravelly, fry, and creak are terms in common use among speech pathologists; yet they mean quite different things to different individuals. Renfrew, Mitchell, and Wallace (1957), working together in a cleft palate team for 4 years assessing speech before and after surgery and speech therapy, set up an experiment in which they listened to recordings and then labelled them independently according to personal judgment. When they came to compare their ratings, they were astonished at the divergence in agreement. They chose five categories of classification: normal resonance, slightly excessive nasal resonance, excessive nasal resonance, insufficient nasal resonance, and mixed resonance. One of the stumbling blocks must have been the category of "nasal escape," which is another possibility and commonly used to denote escape of unvibrated air down the nose.

A universally accepted classification of voice disorders would be a great advantage, for speech therapists could be sure they were talking about the same things. They could be accurate in assessment and progress reports, especially when comparing therapeutic strategies and their failures and successes. Wynter and Martin (1981) spent 5 years in a brave attempt at creating a scientific classification that they could train a captive audience of speech therapy students to remember and use by listening to sample recordings. The categories of dysphonia were selected from 100 voice samples, which a number of qualified therapists listened to and classified in agreement. The categories chosen were: creaky, husky, hoarse, harsh, disordered pitch, disordered resonance, and "others." The "others" category included voices that "defied any attempt to be categorised under existing terminology" (p. 205). This admission at the outset boded ill for the success of a project aimed at laying down a verbal blueprint! The results of this research project proved disappointing, for the auditory perceptions of the trained students failed to match sufficiently closely the perceptions of the researchers. Moreover, it was reported that the students became bored by the project. As Aronson (1980) observes so sensibly, faced with a dysphonia, the clinician's chief concern is diagnosis, not aesthetic values.

Laver (1980) approached the problem from a different angle and endeavored to establish a phonetic description of voice quality by charting the positions of labial, mandibular, lingual, velopharyngeal, and laryngeal structures, to which he gave tension ratings. Phonation type was examined and reduced to categories of harshness, whispery, breathiness, creaky, falsetto, and modal. Laver hoped that by writing a book on these lines and producing a casette would render all clear but soon found that he had to hold seminars to train speech therapists to his ways of thinking. The Laver vocal profile analysis protocol presents a quite formidable list of items and only serves to highlight the enormity of the problems involved and the immense variety of vocal qualities and phonetic gestures possible. The charting of phonetic positions, moreover, was based on observation and listening, mostly conjectures, in fact, and not supported by lateral x-ray photography or xeroradiography (Berry et al., 1982).

# Instruments in Vocal Assessment

There is nowadays a wealth of sophisticated electronic acoustic equipment available to speech scientists and clinicians that renders accurate measurements of certain aspects of voice possible (Cooper, 1973). Accurate information concerning volume, pitch, intonation, and duration of air flow can be displayed on screens showing the original condition and progress during treatment. This equipment can also be used with biofeedback techniques in vocal rehabilitation. The spectrograph and oscilloscope are such instruments (Beckett, 1971; Cooper, 1974; Holbrook, Rolnick, & Bailey, 1974). Pitch meters and volume meters have long been in use also. However, so far no instrument can adequately present the whole picture of an impaired voice and replace the eyes and ears of the speech clinician.

The Kay sonograph held great promise for recording and analyzing resonance. It was hoped that the problem of nasal resonance categories mentioned above could be settled finally. However, the spectrograph registers an embarrassment of frequencies, many of which are redundant to the human ear (Van den Berg, 1962). It is so accurate that it shows how a vowel uttered by the same person contains different frequency components each time it is uttered. The human ear ignores such redundant information and selects (for it) the most pronounced characteristics. Nevertheless, spectrographic analysis in an individual case of hoarseness can be valuable (Cooper, 1974).

The laryngograph (Abberton & Fourcin, 1972; Fourcin, 1981) allows continuous monitoring of vocal cord movement from electrodes placed on either side of the thyroid cartilage. Direct displays of fundamental frequency and amplitude and abnormal shifts and breaks in the LX wave form are registered. The laryngograph can be used to display fundamental frequency derived from the LX wave form on an oscilloscope screen, which is the basis of the Voiscope (Fourcin & Abberton, 1977). The fundamental frequency patterns (intonation) can remain on the Voiscope for as long as needed, and visual feedback of a patient's faulty intonation can be matched to improved patterns and corrected using biofeedback techniques.

A more recent development of considerable interest and value is the xeroradiographic technique developed by Berry et al. (1982). Lateral views of the vocal tract are photographed in life size showing clearly the edge enhancement of soft tissues in three-dimensional depth as well as the contours of bones and cartilages seen in ordinary x-ray photography. For the first time, what speech therapists think they can hear and visualize in the mind's eye can be actually seen in the photographs of dysphonic patients (Julian, MacCurtain, & Noscoe, 1981). Humping of the tongue, lowering of the palate, constriction of the pharynx, elevation of the larynx, the edges of the vocal folds, and intrusion of the ventricular bands are outlined. The photographs can be shown to patients and the abnormal articulatory and vocal antics demonstrated. This reinforces rehabilitation techniques in reducing muscular tension and increasing relaxation.

Respirometery is another useful measure of vocal function, measuring the flow of breath by volume against time. It can be used in diagnosis and as a simple clinical tool in the speech clinic (Amerman & Williams, 1979; Beckett, 1971).

Electronic equipment is expensive, but if funds are available, the most valuable instrument to the speech clinician is probably the Kay Visipitch, which offers the possibility of accurate acoustic analysis of several vocal parameters. It is a reliable diagnostic and biofeedback tool for display of fundamental pitch, intonation, intensity, stress, and duration, with many extra possibilities for imaginative therapy. The Fourcin laryngograph can now be coupled to the Kay Visipitch, which further extends the latter's use as a clinical tool.

# Classification of Voice Disorders

Assessment of vocal quality and function of the vocal instrument is the particular concern of speech pathologists. But in focusing upon vocal symptoms we must not forget fundamental etiology. Classification of dysphonia depends upon the medical diagnosis, without which no responsible therapist will undertake treatment of a patient. Vocal deterioration is frequently the first sign of incipient illness. Dysphonia covers a wide spectrum of physical dysfunction that ranges from simple misuse of the voice to such things as frank neurological disease and surgical intervention in the case of malignancy. The description of voice disorders below follows classification based accordingly upon the priority of medical etiology and not vocal symptomology.

## Vocal Strain (Hyperkinetic Dysphonia)

By far the most common voice disorder is due to poor voice production, which tires the laryngeal mechanism and can even damage the vocal cord surfaces. As already explained, the efficient voice or laryngeal note is dependent upon maintenance of a perfect equilibrium between expiratory pressure and glottal tension. The basic requisite for this is muscular relaxation so that only those muscles required to approximate the vocal cords and control tension (the adductors and tensors) are brought into play as needed. The muscles of respiration must be correctly controlled so that an adequate flow of air from the lungs through the glottis is maintained under steady pressure. When the supply of expired air for phonation (phonic air) is inadequate or erratic, greater force is required to expel air through the glottis to vibrate the cords and obtain adequate volume. The natural pitch is altered at the same time, and resonance and projection of the voice are accordingly impaired. The voice is forced and hard, lacking vibrato. Breathing tends to be upper thoracic or clavicular.

The strain produces an aching throat and is especially felt at the end of the day by inveterate chatterboxes, lecturers, and teachers. This condition, which is very common, is described by speech pathologists as hyperkinetic dysphonia because of the excessive muscular tension involved. In some cases after much strain a hypokinetic condition appears. The vocal muscles exhibit fatigue, weakness, and decreased efficiency, and the cords may appear slack with slight bowing; the voice is feeble and breathy. In all cases there is considerable anxiety, and the psychosomatic aspect must not be undervalued. The vocal strain is frequently exacerbated by domestic worries, pressure at work, or other stressful circumstances. Frequently vocal deterioration follows an attack of influenza and inflammation of the throat and larynx, in which the voice can be temporarily impaired. After such an illness, the delicate vocal mechanism may appear fully recovered, but functionally it remains debilitated and may deteriorate rapidly if overexercised too soon.

The voice may become habitually hoarse, frequently accompanied by a persistent redness of the laryngeal mucosa that is not painful, as in acute infective laryngitis, but is a positive symptom of vocal strain. Irregularity in the vibration of the vocal cords is observable in these hoarse individuals (Dunker & Schlosshauer, 1964). Any unusual vocal symptoms following illness, or occurring at any time, should be investigated by a laryngologist. Once the possibility of disease has been ruled out, speech therapy can commence.

Attention to the general health of the patient is advisable as a first step. Suggestions for alleviating fatigue or stress by better programming the work load are often helpful, along with a discussion of rest, recreation, and diet. A wide variety of social and health activities are available that can help the individual avoid worry, overwork, overeating, and smoking.

Another important step at the commencement of therapy is to explain to the patient exactly what is wrong with voice production and what program for recovery is recommended. Secondly, having located the conditions and situations in which strain is most heavily imposed on the voice, the therapist and patient must plan ways and means for voice conservation. There is no need for total vocal rest; the patient can continue with his or her normal occupations, but for a period should talk quietly—only when strictly necessary and especially not in noisy environments.

Asking the patient to rest the voice totally imposes a great strain and can aggravate gloom and anxiety. Advising the patient not to speak but write everything down is also unwise. Recommending whispering is bad advice, too, because this may damage the vocal cords as much as talking aloud. In strong and forced whispering the vocal cords may be repeatedly adducted in midline and air forced

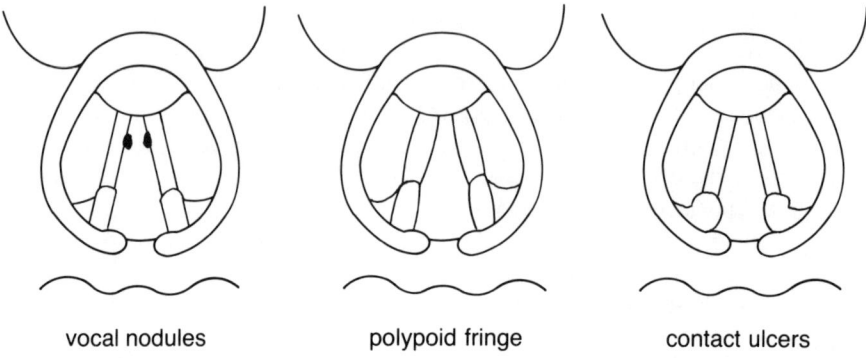

vocal nodules     polypoid fringe     contact ulcers

**Figure 5.** Vocal abuse.

through the triangular aperture between the vocal processes of the arytenoid cartilages.

## Vocal Abuse

Vocal abuse is an advanced stage of vocal strain. Misuse of the voice can be such that friction occurs between the opposing edges and surfaces of the vocal cords. Habitual abuse of the voice causes trauma leading to the formation of vocal nodes, polyps, edema, and occasionally contact ulcers (see Figure 5).

Vocal nodes are one manifestion of vocal abuse. When the vocal cords are forced together with constant hard attack and muscular tension, a localized hemorrhage can develop in a blood vessel. In a single incident such as a loud shout or even an operatic aria this can happen as an isolated event which, with no recurrence of abuse, will disperse and the cords and voice recover. But if vocal abuse becomes habitual, permanent changes take place in the cord surfaces with fibrosis and the formation of nodules. These can be unilateral but generally face each other bilaterally and are sometimes called "kissing nodes" or singer's nodes. The site of occurrence is diagnostic, being at the middle portion of the anterior two thirds of the cords where their maximum excursion is greatest (Luchsinger & Arnold, 1965). They can be quite small or the size of peppercorns.

Depending upon the degree of obstruction impeding approximation of the cords in phonation, the voice will be hoarse, breathy, or aphonic. Small soft nodes will disperse with voice therapy and reduction of hyperfunction, but fibrosed and long-established nodes require surgical removal.

After surgical removal, the cords are quite normal in appearance. Damage does not occur from the instruments of the skilled surgeon. The microlaryngoscopy and endolaryngeal techniques pioneered by Kleinsasser (1968) guarantee success. A patient is generally kept in the hospital a couple of days, and speaking should be avoided during this period. The small ruptures in the epithelium heal rapidly. Zilstorff (1968) recommends a week's complete vocal rest in the case of professional singers, but not longer. Prolonged vocal rest can lead to flaccidity of the vocal muscles, supporting the views of physiotherapists that muscles should be immobilized for the shortest possible time.

Vocal nodes produce a feeling of something in the throat that must be shifted by throat clearing and coughing. This habit may continue after removal of nodes and, as this causes laryngeal abuse, must be corrected. Speech therapy should be prescribed after surgery to prevent recurrence of vocal nodes.

Vocal nodes are more common in children, especially boys. In the British Isles they are a rare occurrence (Greene, 1980) but frequent in the United States, Australia, and New Zealand. This is probably due to the climate and better opportunities for outdoor recreation, whether on the streets or sports grounds. European weather is often more conducive to sitting indoors watching television. The child's activities need to be investigated and evaluated. A solitary small child may play with toy cars, airplanes, and tractors, imitating their engine noises. This may be the cause of the child's vocal nodes, even when parents assure the therapist that the child is quiet and not at all boisterous (Landes, 1977). Many investigators emphasize the psychosomatic aspect of vocal nodes in children (Toohill, 1975; Wilson, 1962, 1977) and point to home problems. Cure is difficult. If the child can follow a voice therapy program and avoid vocal abuse, the prognosis is good. Toohill's study of 77 children reported that, with the help of social workers and parent counselling, only 28 were cured, a success rate similar to that achieved by speech therapists and one that is far from satisfactory. If a child is motivated by a desire to produce a good voice for some purpose such as singing in a choir or acting in a play, therapy can prove effective.

Many New Zealand laryngologists, overwhelmed by the numbers of hoarse children referred to them by school teachers, do not recommend speech therapy and certainly do not remove the nodes surgically unless they are so large that the voice is lost. They simply reassure all involved that nodes are nonmalignant, are due to vocal abuse, and will disappear as the children grow up and shout less. Moreover, as the larynx of the boy grows in puberty and the cords double in length, the pitch drops and the point of maximum excursion of the cords alters position. In most cases the nodes are small and soft and rapidly disperse if given a chance.

Singer's nodes are another sign that the voice has been abused. Vocal nodules do not form on the vocal cords of trained singers, though it is perfectly possible among the best of opera singers for a minute hemorrhage to occur during an exacting role (Punt, 1967). If the opera company's laryngologist administers instant medication, it disperses rapidly. On the other hand, singers of pop and rock, who often use the maximum volume of voice and whose voices are seldom trained, damage their vocal cords frequently and as a result terminate their careers early.

Not uncommonly, the whole edge of one or both cords may be thickened or present a polypoid fringe (see Figure 5). In some singers the peculiar admired quality of the singing voice, such as voice breaks and double notes, is attributable to changes that have taken place in the cords, and therefore should not be corrected surgically until aphonia is actually threatened (Greene, 1980). The voice therapist should be responsible for the rehabilitiation program immediately following surgery. Vocal rest may be maintained for a week or more, and singing practice and engagements banned for some months. Instruction in relaxation and breath control should start at once, and the singer counselled in vocal hygiene. Excessive smoking, smoky atmospheres, and straight alcohol must be avoided. The voice can be rested by avoiding talking against the background noise of restaurants and parties as well as talking too much in the course of ordinary activities. When the larynx has recovered and the singer's speaking voice perfected, he or she should be referred to a competent singing instructor whose teaching of breathing technique is based on sound anatomical and physiological facts.

The polyp, like the vocal node, is a benign neoplasm. There is considerable confusion in the literature regarding the true nature of the vocal fold polyp and the difference between it and a node. Härma, Sonninen, Vartiainen, Haveri, and Väisänen (1975) suggest that nodes and polyps are just different stages in the same process of vocal abuse. Since the location ahd histology are appreciably different, this hypothesis seems ill founded, especially as Kleinsasser (1968) states that their development is completely obscure. He further asserts that in many cases there does not appear to be a history of vocal exertion, though there does in others. Vaughan and Strong (1983) distinguish between sessile polyps (which resemble Reinke's edema but occur unilaterally) and pedunculated polyps (which are associated with vocal abuse).

Kleinsasser (1968) describes several histological types of polyp, the most common being a gelatinous, soft, translucent structure and a fibrous type that may be an advanced stage of the former. The majority occur singly, and the typical location is just behind the anterior commisure on the subglottic surface of the cord. Surgical removal is necessary.

Recommending a program of voice therapy should depend on whether vocal abuse is present. The development of a large polyp causes hoarseness, coughing, and choking, and the interference with phonation can give rise to vocal strain or mechanical overexertion. There is no evidence that inflammatory laryngitis or irritants cause polyps. Luchsinger and Arnold (1965) are definite in their belief that vocal abuse is the cause, and this view is widely accepted. After polypectomy, speech therapy is prescribed by most laryngologists. It is of interest that in the study of Härma et al. (1975) 10 patients who continued to be hoarse after polypectomy were found to be suffering from vocal nodules.

Polypoid fringe (Reinke's edema) is a polypoid degeneration or fringe that may cover the whole length of the vocal cord and is associated with edematous swelling. There is a space between the epithelium covering the muscles and ligaments of the elastic vocal muscle that is occupied by loose connective tissue. This is called Reinke's space, which, when subjected to acute laryngitis and vocal abuse, can fill with fluid. The voice deepens considerably on account of the increased bulk of the vocal cords. Sonninen, Damsté, and Fokkens (1972) suggest that in vocal abuse there is not only friction between the opposing surfaces of the cords but also pulling of the muscles on the ligaments both longitudinally and laterally.

The swelling in Reinke's edema is bilateral and symmetrical and therefore distinguishable from polypoid swelling. The condition may be associated with sinusitis. Kleinsasser (1968) observed that it occurred most commonly among heavy smokers over 40 years of age. Vaughan and Strong (1983) state that edema occurs chiefly among middle-aged women who are heavy smokers and have a long history of vocal abuse and a deep masculine voice. Patients must give up smoking as well as undergo vocal rehabilitation.

Drainage of Reinke's edema is achieved surgically by stripping the vocal cords. The excision is made along the under surface of the one cord and the upper surface of the other in order to avoid adhesion of the raw surfaces in healing. Absolute vocal rest for a week after the operation is advisable. It takes some 3 weeks for healing to be complete, during which time the voice should be used as little as possible. The voice should become normal, and there should be no remaining irregularity of the vocal cords after microsurgery. In some instances, despite successful healing of the epithelium, the voice may remain hoarse and tire readily for some months. This may be due to damage to the mechanoreceptor timing mechanism described by Wyke (1969; 1974). In most cases the cords return to their white healthy appearance and there is a marked rise in vocal pitch. Fritzell, Sunberg, and Strange-Ebbesen (1982) recommend a course of speech therapy *before* stripping the cords so that, in patients showing signs of vocal abuse, there is less risk of trauma when the voice is used after surgery.

Contact ulcers are another symptom of vocal abuse. They form over the posterior portions of the vocal cords and were first described by Jackson and Jackson (1935), who likened the arytenoids to a hammer and anvil striking each other during phonation. The surface of one vocal process is raised and the other slightly hollowed. Ulceration does not actually occur, but keratosis piles up in the cuplike depression. Surgical removal of the granuloma used to be considered necessary (Peacher & Hollinger, 1947). More recently, Peacher (1961) demonstrated that speech rehabilitation was essential, and Vaughan and Strong (1983) do not think surgical removal is advisable. The condition is entirely due to vocal abuse, and the best chance of cure is voice reeducation.

Symptoms of contact ulcers include a painful throat and shooting pains in the ear. The voice has a deep hoarse and hollow quality that is readily identifiable. Almost exclusively a male complaint, contact ulcers are apparently common in the United States but rare in Europe, which would seem to indicate that they are a cultural phenomenon. The patient needs to examine his or her attitude to the voice carefully and cultivate a real desire to improve voice and raise pitch. Hearing training that involves listening to recordings and contrasting the dysphonic voice with the normal male or female voice is helpful. Reduction in laryngeal and pharyngeal tension by methods described below and supporting a smooth vocal note with adduction of the arytenoids and vibration of the pars vocalis of the anterior cords has to be established. Cooper and Nahum (1971) and Peacher (1961) have described detailed methods of vocal rehabilitation. Cure of contact ulcers is a long and difficult process in most cases.

Intubation granuloma, bilateral ulceration of the vocal cords over the arytenoid processes, can be caused by trauma from intralaryngeal intubation for administration of anesthesia during surgical operations. In this case vocal abuse is not the cause, and vocal rest should be prescribed until the ulcers have healed.

# Management of Hyperkinetic Dysphonia

## The Laryngological Report

The first step for a speech pathologist in taking responsibility for the treatment of any dysphonic patient is to obtain and study the otolaryngologist's report. The condition of the larynx and the vocal cords will be described based on direct or indirect laryngoscopy and sometimes fiberoptic endoscopy. Hearing will have been tested and general health checked either by the laryngologist or by the referring general practitioner. The prescription of drugs, especially tranquilizers, should be known. An experienced laryngologist with an interest in voice disorders can give the voice therapist valuable guidance in diagnosis and support during treatment. If possible, the speech pathologist should view the patient's larynx over the shoulder of the laryngologist, which, though not essential, is often a revelation. Some American speech pathologists are accustomed to carrying out indirect laryngoscopy themselves, but the medically unqualified voice therapist in many other parts of the world prefers not to take on this responsibility. Hoarseness and inflammation of the cords can be a symptom of several problems: bacterial infection, vocal strain, or a malignancy.

## The Case History

The great majority of speech pathologists have to work without the assistance of an acoustic laboratory or any of the electroacoustic instruments described above. They have to rely upon their own training and experience in taking a case history as well as their eyes and ears in judging the type and cause of dysphonia. Information relevant to the voice is gathered by skillful questioning. Further details may emerge in subsequent sessions as the patient gains insight into his or her condition and confidence in the therapist. The first interview is important. It is necessary to establish a friendly but professional relationship from the outset. An apparently unsympathetic comment may lose a touchy patient's full cooperation, in which case the prognosis regarding speech rehabilitation is not promising.

The patient's complaints and attitude to the voice problem need to be heard. The duration of hoarseness and events leading up to its development are noted down.

The conditions at home and work also need to be examined. Is a factory, office, school, or home too noisy? Is it necessary to talk too much? Can circumstances be ameliorated? Often the actual cause of damage is other than what first seems obvious.

A head teacher complaining of hoarseness was found to be suffering from the first signs of vocal nodules upon indirect laryngoscopy. He certainly was tense, a shallow breather, with a tendency to shout and gesticulate, but he had done very little teaching for the past 6 months, performing administrative work instead. He did not agree that he suffered from vocal strain and was convinced he had throat cancer. Upon careful questioning and only after the third interview, it was revealed that the teacher travelled to and from the city on a noisy train in the company of friends to whom he talked for approximately 2 hours a day. Voice therapy, restoration of teaching duties, and reading on the train effected a cure.

A cash register assistant in a supermarket, seated in the usual position near the exit doors and street traffic, would not be expected to develop vocal nodules while attending to her duties but was found to talk incessantly to customers and to shout to colleagues beside her down the line.

Irritants such as dust, smoke, alcohol, and an overly dry atmosphere due to central heating or air conditioning can perpetuate chronic laryngitis and contribute to vocal strain. Shouting at deaf relatives and at children can impair the voice.

In most cases patients exhibit anxieties and stress engendered by domestic or occupational tensions. Effective therapy must include sympathy, understanding, acceptance, and encouragement to talk out problems while contributing practical suggestions and solutions. The speech pathologist helps put facts into focus and presents all sides of a question confronting the patient, which he or she might tend to overlook in an irrational preoccupation with some details (Rippon & Fletcher, 1940).

Close collaboration with the laryngologist must be maintained throughout treatment and periodic review of the larynx requested. Other workers may be called in: parents and teachers of children with vocal nodes, social workers, personnel and employment officers in the case of adults. Patients suffering from serious emotional disturbance should be referred to a psychiatrist, but by and large the experienced otolaryngologist does not refer such patients for vocal rehabilitation.

## Voice and Speech Recording

A recording should be made at the first interview. It will be of value as a referral point in subsequent treatment and rehabilitation. Often a patient will be depressed at slow progress but encouraged by hearing how the voice sounded previously—before treatment started. The recording should include a sample of conversation, a short passage of reading, prolonged vowel sounds, and some mechanical material such as counting aloud on one breath or reciting days of the week.

A simple explanation of how the patient is misusing the voice and an outline of the rehabilitation program must be given. The first interview should also include a brief demonstration of how to breathe and relax and suggestions for putting new ideas into practice. Thus the individual is given something constructive to do and can feel that the road is open to recovery.

Voice therapy sessions should be arranged ideally twice or three times in the first week after the preliminary interview. This gives the patient a chance to master relaxation and diaphragmatic breathing quickly in practice periods to alleviate excessive vocal strain. Then weekly sessions can be arranged over a period of a month or two as required. It takes time to establish the habits of normal voice production in everyday conversation.

## Clinical Assessment of the Dysphonic Patient

It is useful to have a simple form available for each patient which serves as a check list so that useful details can be jotted down quickly (see Figure 6). It is all too easy in a busy day to forget to ask for items such as a telephone number and home doctor, or to think one will remember details later.

# Rehabilitation for Hyperkinetic Dysphonia

Vocal rehabilitation procedures are based on fundamental principles of normal voice production. Even in cases when the vocal instrument is irreparably impaired and changed by disease and/or surgery, as in laryngectomy, the basic principles still apply. The voice therapist must constantly compare normal with abnormal function and decide how best to adapt exercises to overcome difficulties and develop the patient's potential within the boundaries imposed by the pathologic etiology.

The next section describes a basic program for voice therapy that can be followed through in the relatively straightforward area of hyperkinetic dysphonia. More difficult types of organic, psychologic, and neurologic dysphonia will then be discussed, each encompassing the adjuncts to the basic scheme to meet the demands of the particular disability.

A monograph such as this is largely a scan of the specialized field of dysphonia, the aim being to understand etiology and therapy and acquire a guide to further exploration. The postgraduate student's competence will be enhanced by careful study of scientific articles and the standard works such as Boone (1977); Brodnitz (1971); Cooper and Cooper (1977); Greene (1980); and Wilson (1979).

## Relaxation

Bodily relaxation reduces tension in the antagonistic muscles and improves coordination or the rhythm and flow of movement. Although relaxation may be induced by tranquilizers, it is desirable for patients to learn to relax by natural means as therapy proceeds. Relaxation induces calm and reduces anxiety.

Many methods are based on suggestion—the conjuring up of visual pictures of tranquility and peace, perhaps reinforced by suitable musical accompaniment. Progressive relaxation may be induced by stretching and flexing limbs and "letting go" (Jacobson, 1934). The patient may sit in a chair or lie on a couch. The therapist tests the joints to be sure ankles, wrists, and neck are loose. Special attention to the head, neck, and shoulders in areas where tension produces

Name _____

Age _____ Date of birth _____

Address _____

Telephone _____

Occupation _____

Referring doctor _____

Diagnosis _____

Medication _____

1. Personality type: high-strung, anxious, aggressive

2. Posture: slouching, stiff military, etc.

3. Tension: general and localized

4. Mannerisms: fidgety, gestures, facial expression, eye contact

5. Breathing at rest and in speech:
    Type—clavicular, abdominal, rapid, irregular
    Control in speech—air wastage, gasping, sighing
    Nasal/oral breathing at rest and in speech

6. Vocal symptoms
    Phonation: hoarse, metallic, gravelly
    Vowel prolongation: hard attack
    Pitch: appropriate/too high/too low
    Inflection: monotonous/exaggerated
    Resonance: nasality/head resonance
    Volume: projection loud/soft

7. Speech: fast/slow/jerky/incoherent

8. Articulation: open/closed/faults/dialect

9. Instruments used and measurements of tests completed

**Figure 6.** Sample case sheet.

rheumatic pains and even headache is required. Children can simulate floppy animals or puppets on strings and are easily suggestible if their imaginations are captivated.

## Breathing

Establishment of intercostal diaphragmatic breathing and correction of upper thoracic, shallow, or rapid respiration is necessary. This may be taught while the patient relaxes on a couch or sits easily in a chair or stands erect, feet apart. Practice in all positions is advisable as correct patterns have to be established in every situation. A good erect posture is important.

Breathing through the mouth on inspiration is necessary when the patient practices speaking. This quick intake of oral breath occurs naturally between words and phrases. The nostrils naturally obstruct rapid inspiration. Controlled expiration is achieved by counting aloud, chanting, uttering prolonged vowels, and humming. If the patient needs to rest the voice or is aphonic, prolonged fricatives and affricates are preferable, especially for home practice. Control of chest movement should be felt with hands on waist.

When the correct breathing pattern comes easily and habitual upper thoracic movement is eradicated, the changed rhythm for speech may be introduced—a quick oral intake of air and prolonged expiration.

## Phonation

Vocal practice and breath control have already opened the way to vocal exercises and further improvement of the voice. Vowels with soft attack must be held steady and clear on the natural speaking pitch of the patient. This pitch may at first be difficult to ascertain in strained voices, but may come quite naturally as relaxation and phonic control increase without strain and tension. Sometimes natural pitch is indicated by the patient's laugh or by humming up and down the scale until optimum resonance is heard and felt, the voice sounding rich in harmonics and strong. Strong chest vibrations may be felt by the fingers in male speakers and vibrations in the nasal and malar bones of females. Vocal flexibility must be gained by exercises in varied patterns of intonation and rhythm. Vocal exercises are necessary in practicing vowels, syllables, and rhymes, and the same sentence can be spoken with different intonation patterns and meaning.

## Listening

Hearing training in contrasting a good vocal note with a poor one, variations in pitch, and projection must be demonstrated by the therapist and imitated by the patient. Tape recordings are very useful, and work at home with a tape recorder to reinforce lessons and allow self-monitoring is valuable.

## Articulation (Diction)

An approach to open articulation will already have been included in developing vowel resonance. Consonants may be indistinct or even faulty, and these should be practiced for clearer definition in syllables, words, and sentences. Just one aberrant consonant, especially an /s/ or /sh/, can mar delivery whereas its eradication can normalize speech and improve self-confidence considerably.

## Froeschels' Chewing Therapy

This specialized form of therapy has never caught on in the British Isles but is popular in Europe, Scandinavia, and the United States, where the Vienna school of speech pathology took root after World War II. Froeschels (1952) described the rationale for the use of chewing exercises for developing vocal relaxation. Chewing is a natural primitive activity involving the speech organs but disassociated from the tensions habitual in the speech of a dysphonic patient. Chewing and vocalizing, producing strings of nonsense syllables (the talk of a savage), permits phonation to take place with relaxed larynx, pharynx, and oral muscles. Through the munching and chumping of nonsense syllables, a relaxed voice with the optimum pitch range can emerge naturally and then be gradually transferred through exercises into speech (Brodnitz, 1971; Froeschels, 1952; Weiss & Beebe, 1951).

## Biofeedback

Displays on screens, if the necessary instrumentation is available, can be used throughout treatment as discussed earlier. Electromyography is used in relaxation. Sound waves portraying pitch, volume, resonance, and duration can be monitored from separate instruments or an acoustic analyzer that incorporates several kinds of instruments such as the Kay Visipitch.

The biofeedback remedial program must be supported by the voice practices described above. The efficacy of biofeedback alone, where patients are left to their own devices and expected to cure themselves, has proved disappointing. Improvement in isolated aspects of speech must be reinforced by work with the therapist so that improved phonation is carried over into conversation in real-life situations (Dalton, 1983). The relationship between patient and therapist must be such that the therapist knows what these real-life situations are and makes rehabilitation a reality, not just a series of exercises.

## Habituation

Normal voice has to become automatic and habitual. The dysphonic patient must reach a stage when relaxation, breathing, phonating, and speaking correctly become second nature. To this end, vocal technique must be established in a range of speech situations—conversation, reading, poetry reading, giving talks, debating, and telephoning. Activities confined at first to the clinical situation must extend to situations familiar to the individual. For example, if the domestic or working environment is polluted with noise, background noise may be provided in the speech clinic by playing suitable recordings while the patient speaks and learns not to tense up and resort to forced phonation.

# Psychological (Functional) Dysphonia

## Anxiety States

Many patients at the otolaryngological clinic who are passed on to the speech therapist for treatment are not suffering from any physical disability and do not even show laryngeal signs of any importance but are victims of mild anxiety states. They complain of vocal weakness or hoarseness coupled with varied symptoms of discomfort in the throat, such as feelings of pressure, aching, a lump, or choking from catarrh. A careful medical examination of patients complaining of these symptoms, often referred to as *globus hystericus*, must be carried out to exclude organic causes. Malcomson (1968) found that, out of 307 patients complaining of a lump in the throat (90 males and 217 females), 38% had miscellaneous local lesions and 62% distal lesions, of which the most common (69%) was hiatus hernia. Osteoarthritis of the cervical spine is a common cause of referred pain. Pressure symptoms can be real, caused by an enlarged thyroid gland. When no organic cause can be found, the feeling of a lump in the throat must be ascribed to psychogenic disorder and treated accordingly.

Linford-Rees (1967) gives multiple factors in the etiology of anxiety states. The intrinsic constitutional makeup of the individual is genetically determined. It may predispose to anxiety, which is aggravated by environmental factors with some particular stress or a series of anxiety-loaded events precipitating breakdown. Anxiety-prone individuals are always apprehensive—expecting the worst, worrying about their health, their family, their work. They are likely to develop psychosomatic symptoms. They are active and tense, restless, and fidgety, with rapid and often incessant speech. Tension in the muscular system produces real aches and pains, and an aching throat can commonly become a focus of attention and worry, especially as speech so often is associated with stressful situations. Cancer phobias are common. With such patients the most important need is a satisfactory and reassuring relationship with the speech pathologist. Great relief is obtained from discussing anxieties and problems that have been too long "bottled up." A trouble shared is indeed a trouble halved. These patients need understanding, sympathy, and support until feelings of security and confidence develop. Although there is little organically wrong with the voice and the throat, it is of no use telling this to these patients because they feel something *is* wrong. It is beneficial to treat the symptoms by a course of relaxation and voice production to run concurrently with the supportive therapy. When the discomfort in the throat is relieved, the patient is led to gain insight into the link between physical sensations and the enviromental stress. Such patients are rewarding to treat. They are often extremely appreciative of the kindness and help given.

## Hysterical Voice Disorders

Hysteria is defined as a psychogenic illness in which the patient manifests certain signs of mental or physical disorder for some real or imagined gain, without being fully aware of the underlying motive. In this respect it is distinct from malingering, in which the individual claims to have symptoms while knowing he or she has none. The hysterical disorder may simulate any illness or disorder. The symptoms conform to the patient's concept of the disease. Hysterical reactions may include disturbances of consciousness (e.g., amnesia and fugues), conversion symptoms of motor paralysis, or sensory loss (e.g., paresthesia, hyperalgesia or pains, blindness, deafness). Visceral disorders include vomiting, constipation, retention of urine, and anorexia. These symptoms are all capable of being produced by volitional processes and conform to the patient's own concept of the disease. They are therefore unlike the manifestations of emotional tension mediated by the autonomous nervous system as occur in anxiety states and psychosomatic disorders.

There is a specific and easily recognized type of hysterical personality (Linford-Rees, 1967). It is not considered to have a familial basis but becomes conditioned by environment. The hysteric needs to exaggerate and dramatize, to be the center of attention, and to create a favorable impression. There is a tendency to manipulate people and situations for personal gain. Emotional reactions and attachments are shallow, and the need to dramatize and exaggerate leads naturally to distortion of the truth, an important aspect to be borne in mind when taking the case history of such people and subsequent reports of incidents. Some have been deprived of affection and have an insatiable desire for approval and affection, which may test those who give to such an extent that they are driven away. Hysteria is a result of anxiety and insecurity, a defense mechanism designed to protect the individual from threats arising out of an inherent inadequacy for dealing with responsibilities.

Hysterical voice disorders may range from total loss of the voice to acquisition of a strange voice for short or long periods due to a functional paralysis of the adductor and tensor muscles of the larynx. Only forced whispering may be possible due to partial failure in adduction of the cords, which adduct along the anterior muscular section but present an open triangle posteriorly. Bowing of the cords ("internal tensor weakness") occurs with poor functioing of the tensor muscles—the voice is weak and breathy or comes and goes. Sometimes there is excessive tension, and an abnormally high pitch or falsetto can be assumed by both males and females, or a double note. In such cases paralysis of vocal muscles is obviously not present, as movements on coughing, breathing, and laughing are normal. The voice may be very bizarre, bearing no resemblance to the patient's real voice. In some instances the ventricular bands approximate toward the midline above the paralyzed vocal cords, producing a raucous, sometimes double-noted sound while the vocal cords are capable of perfectly normal approximation.

Response to voice therapy is affected by the duration and severity of the personality disturbance. A patient who comes from an unstable family and has shown personality instability since childhood, developing illness to avoid responsibility or unpleasant situations, may recover normal voice but relapse constantly or develop any of the other conversion symptoms mentioned above. An acute onset of voice disorder following really traumatic incidents in persons of relative stability have a better prognosis. These are the patients with whom the speech pathologist can succeed and thus relieve the psychiatrist's load. It is generally agreed that the symptom should be cured quickly and, if at all possible, at the first session. Patients should not be allowed to think it is serious or worthy of much attention. Firmness and suggestion should be combined along with every effort to make patients assume responsibility for cure.

Vocal exercises, vowels with hard attack, and jerking the arms down from the elbows may be given for aphonia or whispering symptoms. Frequently, if the voice does not return, patients are told it will return the next day if practice continues, and it generally does. Certain pitch variations may respond to vowels based on a cough or laugh, which are generally normal. The rapport established with the therapist while taking the case history is all-important—patients should gain the impression that difficulties are understood and that courage in carrying on despite the vocal affliction is admirable, but even more admirable will be the recovery of voice. Supportive therapy may be continued for a period when the patient is helped to cope with difficulties. But the patient should be discharged before vocal symptoms recur and the patient becomes too dependent upon the therapist. If the patient fails to respond to voice therapy, it should not be allowed to continue, and the patient should be referred to a psychiatrist, who can employ far more powerful tactical aids such as hypnosis and intravenous barbituate narcosis.

## The Hyperventilation Syndrome

It is widely accepted in psychological medicine that anxiety and breathing disorder are highly correlated (Lewis, 1959). In recent years attention has been drawn to a particular type of ventilation in anxiety that becomes a chronic feature and sparks off panic attacks in stressful situations. Lum (1976) has been the pioneer in drawing attention to the hyperventilation syndrome. The consequence of rapid clavicular breathing is to produce arterial hypocapnia. The drop in the level of carbon dioxide in the blood is reflected also in the level in alveolar air. This is measurable with a capnograph, which, by a nonintrusive technique, sucks in the breath of a subject and instantly analyzes each expiration, measuring the carbon dioxide output in the end tidal air. It also records the breathing rate per minute, which should be between 8 cpm and 12 cpm in normals at rest and is an important diagnostic sign.

Lowering of the carbon dioxide level affects most bodily systems and gives rise to symptoms of disease where none actually exists. Diseases simulated may be cardiovascular, neurologic, respiratory, muscular-skeletal, gastrointestinal, and psychological (Hardonk & Beumer, 1979; Lewis, 1959; Magarian, 1983).

An individual who is a chronic hyperventilator and subject to all sorts of strange symptoms may suffer attacks of panic in certain situations and be so afraid of recurrence of the psychosomatic symptoms that a conditioned reflex habit develops. Lum (1976), observing that panic is accompanied by disordered breathing, evolved a method of breathing training by which the patient learns to inhibit attacks (Innocenti, 1983). Lum (1981) claimed that in a sample of over 1,000 patients, 95% were cured or much improved by simply retraining breathing. However, this finding has been questioned by medical specialists following up Lum's work and seeking confirmation by controlled trials and objective measurements (Hibbert, 1984).

Hyperventilation has so many different symptoms that a patient can be referred to practically any department of a general hospital. Complaints cannot be considered lightly and need investigation because they may indicate real disease and also because hyperventilation can coexist with asthma or a heart condition. Bass and Gardner (1984) have written an excellent survey of the problem. Diagnosis is difficult, but, when arrived at, management may include drugs that reduce palpitations, trembling, and sweating as well as raise the $pCO_2$ and treat anxiety. Breathing training from a physiotherapist and behavior therapy for phobias from a psychologist can be prescribed.

Greene, Timmons, and Glover (1983; 1984), impressed by the resemblance of some symptoms exhibited by patients diagnosed as suffering from functional hysterical conversion dysphonia and those of hyperventilators, carried out a pilot study of six patients being treated by speech therapists. Two patients were diagnosed as hyperventilators using a capnograph and a provocation test of voluntary rapid breathing. Their histories also supported diagnoses of hyperventilation syndrome. Common symptoms are dizziness, tingling or numb extremities, fears, throat discomfort, clavicular breathing, and frequent sighing and yawning. The study confirmed the supposition that hyperventilation is a factor to be taken into account in dysphonia and a syndrome that speech therapists should be able to recognize. Traditional breathing training in the diaphragmatic method, relaxation and transfer into speaking, and sympathetic counseling are not only suitable but altogether necessary (Greene, 1984). It is questionable, however, that this therapy will alone bring about a cure. The two patients diagnosed had been attending the speech clinic for a long period without notable improvement in voice production. A psychiatric assessment was indicated but actually rejected by the patients. Ideally with such patients the speech therapist needs to hand over these cases to a psychiatrist and psychologist entirely or work very closely with them.

# Systemic Disorders

## Spastic Dysphonia

Spastic dysphonia (spasmodic adductor dysphonia) is a complex and perplexing voice disorder of unknown etiology but clear symptomology. It is characterized by adductor spasms of the vocal cords that are most conspicuous in the production of vowel sounds. The voice is produced with excessive effort and is described as "strangulated." It often develops after an acute viral laryngitis and/or psychological trauma and is incurable. Aronson (1973) has produced a publication with audiocassettes illustrating cases of functional dysphonia. The many examples of spastic dysphonia are invaluable study for speech pathologists unfamiliar with the vocal symptoms.

Symptoms vary in severity, becoming less severe during "good" spells and more severe under stress. A significant feature is that the voice often improves remarkably with a change of speech pathologist, doctor, or psychiatrist. This led to acceptance of the view that the disorder was a psychogenic or hysterical manifestation (Arnold & Heaver, 1959). But views on this etiology have changed since Robe, Brumlik, and Moore (1960) reported abnormal EEGs in 10 cases of spastic dysphonia and Aronson, Brown, Litin, and Pearson (1968a) reported the presence of associated neurologic tremor of tongue, head, and hand in 20 out of 34 cases of spastic dysphonia. Evidence of central neurologic impairment involving the cranial nerves is accumulating, but the fact that many cases have no neurological signs at all still leaves much room for speculation.

Schaeffer (1983) has reported the results of an exhaustive examination of spasmodic dysphonia patients to establish neurologic etiology. Three parameters of brain-stem function were tested: auditory, gastric, and cardiac pathways. A significant correlation was found between central nervous system impairment and vocal tremor. Schaeffer (1983) speculates that the wide spectrum of disability and the fact that some sufferers have no other neurologic signs represent different stages in cranial nerve deterioration. He noted stabilization of the condition over a period of 3 to 5 years. Slow progression or even arrest of impairment in some cases would account for those cases, often erroneously diagnosed as functional and treated for considerable periods by speech pathologists. This is not at all inappropriate management, for patients adapt and learn to live with their disability, perhaps a better solution in the long run than surgical intervention, which often leads to relapse.

Voice therapy, though not a cure, is very helpful, and Greene (1980) reported the beneficial results in many patients receiving treatment in India. Remedial work must concentrate on relaxation, breathing technique, and phonation with a soft, breathy vocal attack to reduce the adductor spasm. The following case note demonstrates the type of spastic dysphonia that benefits from voice therapy (Greene, Timmons, & Glover, 1983). A man 55 years old had suffered from hoarseness for 6 years, which after some changes in speech pathologists was diagnosed as spastic dysphonia. At the time of onset he had married not very happily for a second time after 10 years of freedom following his divorce. He was cheerful and happy and enjoyed attention. A normal voice appeared now and then in conversation, and he was able to produce isolated vowels normally. He could also sing with no audible tremor. Fiberoptic exploration showed a relaxed pharynx and normal movement of the vocal cords. Altogether he presented a picture of functional dysphonia, except that he could not be cured and he had good and bad periods—indicating perhaps a slow progression of neurologic impairment or an arrest in neurologic deterioration.

## Recurrent Laryngeal Nerve Section

In 1967 Dedo (1976) was confronted by a desperate female patient who had been seeking specialists' advice for 17 years, refusing to accept her condition of spastic dysphonia. He decided to experiment with paralyzing one vocal cord with an injection of lidocaine, reasoning that this would alleviate the symptom of overadduction of the cords. The experiment provided instant relief of the vocal symptoms, which warranted the further step of performing a recurrent laryngeal nerve section. The voice produced was breathy, but it improved with speech therapy (Dedo & Lawson, 1977).

Since then, laryngologists have performed many hundreds of recurrent laryngeal nerve sections. After operation the voice may not be normal, although it gives great relief from struggle symptoms in phonation. Patients should be warned of this and be given an opportunity to hear recordings of their speech during the mandatory lidocaine test. Some patients, probably those with a predominance of psychogenic disorder, express dissatisfaction with the result and refuse surgery.

Unfortunately it has been found that all too frequently the voice improvement is not maintained and overadduction by the healthy cord achieves spasmodic contact with the paralyzed cord (Lawrence, 1979). The patient is disappointed but not surprised if warned of the possibility beforehand. In all cases patients maintain that it is easier to speak than it was before surgery and appear reasonably satisfied. Some laryngologists may suggest nerve section of the unoperated cord, but this seems fraught with risk; it is better to rely on voice therapy.

Dedo and Shipp (1980) have suggested that the cause of recurrence of spastic dysphonia is the habitual striving for greater vocal volume. They recommend speech therapy after nerve section for all patients. Fritzell, Feuer, Haglund, Knutsson, & Schiratzki (1982) reported on the postoperative progress of four patients, two of whom suffered from recurrence of spasm. They believe that the sectioned nerve reinervates because electromyographic records clearly showed intermittent bursts of energy in the operated side. A further interesting observation in this report is the fact that the two cases who relapsed vocally were the two who did not have a course of speech therapy postoperatively.

## Dysphonia as a Result of Psychiatric Chemotherapy

A note on the effects of drugs upon the voice is appropriate as a corollary to the preceding section. The voice therapist should inquire whether the patient has been on any prescription drugs that may be responsible for voice disorder. There are widely disparate reactions to drugs; some people can tolerate large doses of one drug without ill effects whereas others develop side effects from small doses. It is not unusual for the otolaryngologist to prescribe a tranquilizer for an anxious patient. It helps the patient to relax and helps speech therapy.

These drugs are mild and have no side effects but are addictive. Drugs given for depression, with an atropine effect, dry up the mouth, throat, and larynx and cause urinary retention. Patients with an induced laryngis sicca develop hoarseness that can erroneously be attributed to nervous disorder. The voice recovers as soon as the drug is withdrawn. Gawel (1981) has provided a valuable review of the effects of various drugs on speech, as has Lee (1983) in connection with stuttering.

Other drugs prescribed for anxiety and depression can produce giddiness, nausea, blurred vision, drowsiness, and forgetfulness. Drug therapy should be checked when hyperventilators are referred for voice and breathing therapy by psychiatrists, an increasing possibility now that this syndrome is better understood.

# Endocrine Disorders

Disturbances in the endocrinological system are closely associated with voice disorders. An extensive and excellent survey of the disorders and types of dysphonia was written by Luchsinger and Arnold (1965). Mutual interdependence of the various endocrine glands is extremely complicated, and many of the problems related to such conditions as hermaphroditism, acromegaly, and precocious vocal mutation are of chiefly academic interest since their treatment is medical. It is possible here to refer to only the more common endocrine disorders that give rise to dysphonia, all of which remain medical problems, of course, but may be misdiagnosed and are quite frequently referred to the speech therapist erroneously as "functional disorders"—that is, attributed to an indeterminate etiology of vocal strain and neurotic traits.

Vocal changes occur as a result of ingestion of the mucous membrane of the larynx during ovarian changes in females. During puberty the voice is often husky and the cords slightly reddened. Singing and overtaxing the voice should be avoided during this period. Some women's voices grow husky during the menstrual period, and singers in particular should not perform if this is so. Hoarseness may appear during pregnancy. The climacteric is another period of vocal instability. Edema of the cords causes deepening of the voice. Excessive smoking and coughing may increase irritation and dysphonia. If the speaker is a professional voice user and has habitually poor voice production, a course of voice therapy may prove very beneficial.

## Myxedema

Thyroid disease frequently affects the voice, and in the early stages of illness voice change may be the first symptom to appear. Undersecretion of the gland, hypothyroidism (which produces cretinism in children), may be acquired late in life. Myxedema of the vocal cords causes an increase in bulk and considerable drop in pitch, which is naturally more conspicuous in women than in men.

Myxedema is comparatively common in the elderly. It is accompanied by gain in weight, thinning hair, and drying of the skin. These signs are natural to the aging process, but, if accompanied by a change of voice encompassing a drop in pitch and a characteristic hollow hoarseness, myxedema can be suspected. Elderly people living alone may not be aware of an insidious deterioration in health, but social workers and other welfare visitors can detect abnormal vocal change in those growing old and exhibiting the signs of slowness and forgetfulness that also accompany myxedema. Treatment with thyroxin will cure the hypothyroidism, but the voice does not generally improve (Heinemann, 1969).

## Thyrotoxicosis

Oversecretion of the thyroid gland causes thyrotoxicosis. The voice may tire easily and be weak or severely hoarse due to compression of the laryngeal nerves by an enlarged gland. Respiration is more rapid in thyrotoxicosis and vital capacity reduced. There is marked nervousness and instability. Sonninen (1960), in an analysis of 131 patients who underwent thyroidectomy, found that a number of them had no thyrotoxicosis in the blood analysis and the only sign was that of compression and a weak voice, especially evident in shouting, which he used as a test. Slight enlargement of the gland may give rise to a feeling of a lump, choking feelings, or vague discomfort in the throat on swallowing, which can easily be attributed to nervous disorder. Because of the excitability and emotional lability of thyrotoxic patients, the female "thyroid syndrome" is always a difficult one to sort out when toxic symptoms and enlargement of the gland are minimal and neurotic traits appear uppermost. Speech therapy and reassurance may alleviate the nervous and vocal symptoms when medication and surgery are deemed unnecessary or inadvisable by the specialist.

## Sexual Immaturity

Disturbance of the sex hormones is another important endocrine cause of voice disorder. Castration in the male before puberty prevents vocal mutation and was common in Europe in the 18th century when the castrati singers or countertenors were popular (Moses, 1960). Pituitary deficiency may prevent development of secondary sexual characteristics and growth of the larynx, resulting in failure of voice break. Maturity in some boys is delayed until the late teens but may develop normally without medication.

## Virilization of the Voice

Among women, development of a deep voice is called virilization of the voice. It can develop as a result of a tumor of the ovaries or adrenal glands that excrete androgens (male hormones). It may occur after administration of testosterone in treatment of gynecological carcinoma. Damsté (1964) drew attention to virilization of the voice due to anabolic steroids. The voice is not hoarse but actually strong and deep. Administration of testosterone is a life-preserving treatment, and voice change is a small price to pay for this. It is a quite different matter when testosterone is given in the treatment of climacteric complaints. Shepperd (1966) describes five cases of women with androgenic hoarseness and increased growth of hair. In all cases the presence of hormones in the prescribed commercial preparations was not suspected by the doctor and was only detected by the laryngologist. Voice change takes months to develop fully. The voice is initially unsteady and wavering between high and low notes, the patient being nervous about speaking until it stabilizes. Singing is impossible. Once the voice has dropped, neither withdrawal from the androgens nor administration of estrogens (female hormones) improves the voice. Changes in the vocal cords are irreversible, but voice therapy may help younger patients to adapt and obtain a new balance between vocal cord tension and phonic pressure.

## Failure in Voice Mutation in Males (Puberphonia)

Failure of the adolescent male to acquire a male voice may be due to endocrinological or structural laryngeal abnormalities. If the development of secondary sexual characteristics proceeds normally, the laryngeal cartilages increase in size with considerable growth in the length of the vocal cords. The pitch of the boy's voice drops an octave and acquires masculine overtones generated by the laryngeal and chest resonators. In some cases the voice fails to break and retains its piping falsetto, or there is a prolonged "stormy mutation" with unpredictable pitch breaks. Sometimes a strange "double note" or pitch fluctuation contributed by the head and chest registers is evident. In the absence of physical causes the symptom is psychogenic. Failure of a mature personality to develop and fear of growing up and assuming the male role and its responsibilities stem from the environment and the boy's relations with his parents. There may be too close a relationship with the mother, who has an overprotective attitude and channels marital frustrations into solicitude for the son. Relations with the father are often found to be unsatisfactory, if not patently antagonistic (Greene, 1980). In some cases the father has left home. The patient is often found to be the only sibling. Effeminacy may be evident. Sometimes the boy's voice has broken prematurely, and being self-conscious among his contemporaries, he has striven to maintain a boy's voice, which has then become habitual. Seth and Guthrie (1935) mention successful boy sopranos who are loathe to drop out of the limelight when their voices break. Weiss (1950) has written a comprehensive account of pubertal voice change.

These patients, when they have a sincere desire to acquire a normal voice, and generally they have if they have got as far as the speech clinic, are not difficult to treat. At the first session, a recording of the patient's effeminate voice should be played back to him; then a deep voice should be elicited, at least on a prolonged vowel, and maintained in counting. Frequently, if pitch breaks are a symptom, the patient is able to speak in his new voice immediately, especially when praised for this fine, masculine voice. The most successful method of establishing deep pitch is from a cough, which is in most cases normal. Singing down the scale, pressing on the cartilage while humming (which relaxes the vocal cords and lowers the pitch), and acting the role of an old man are all effective methods. A psychiatrist should be consulted if the reauired voice is not produced and maintained soon.

Attention to improving voice production as well as confidence may be necessary, especially if there is much habitual laryngeal tension and shallow or upper thoracic breathing and the boy is going to teach or adopt any profession making demands upon his voice.

If the boy is still in his teens, his mother, and if possible, his father should be interviewed and given some counsel. Rehabilitation should encourage the boy to be independent and increase his circle of friends, male and female, and social and sports activities.

# Structural Anomalies and Abnormalities

## Insufficient Nasality (Hyponasality)

A deflected septum causes nasal obstruction and reduces nasality besides rendering nose-breathing difficult. The condition is commonly caused by fracture of the nasal bones in accidents (Gross & Johnson, 1977). Congenital abnormalities of nasal bones and deflected septum are also frequent in cleft palate. A neoplasm or polyp may occur in patients subject to allergic rhinitis.

The most prevalent cause of nasal obstruction and insufficient nasality is met in children with hypertrophy of tonsils and adenoids. The voice may be hoarse from frequent colds and laryngitis. In these cases medication or surgery is the first course of action. When the nose and throat are clear and healthy, speech should be normal, but nose-blowing and resonance exercises may be necessary to correct bad habits (Greene, 1980). An audiological assessment is advisable.

Resonance exercises will require hearing training contrasting nasal and denasalized speech, followed by humming. Feeling the buzzing sounds beneath fingertips placed on the nasal bones as well as feeling vibrations (tingling) of the lips are useful exercises. Practice of words composed of vowels and nasal consonants, introduction of these words into phrases, and rhymes stressing nasal resonance will help the transfer of normal resonance into a child's speech.

## Hearing Loss

Infected adenoids may obstruct the eustachian tubes, causing blurred hearing and intermittent hearing loss following the course of infection. The effect on a young child developing speech will be considerable and may go unnoticed. A high proportion of children with delayed speech and language have early histories of throat infection and ear trouble and many are retarded at school in reading and writing. This may also be due to frequent absences from school. Hearing will of course be checked by an audiologist before and after treatment for enlarged adenoids, but the educational handicap of early hearing impairment must be investigated. School progress should be examined and, if necessary, extra instruction arranged to enable the child to catch up.

## Excessive Nasality (Hypernasality)

Excessive nasality is most commonly due to unsuccessfully repaired cleft palate, undetected submucous cleft, a short palate, or a deep pharynx, which may not become evident until after adenoidectomy. The primary problem is the choice of suitable plastic surgery and/or prosthodontia, followed by voice training to eradicate nasality if necessary (Bernstein, 1979).

The assessment of velopharyngeal function, when primary repair of cleft palate has failed, requires sophisticated methods carried out in specialized plastic surgery clinics (Pigott, 1983; Pigott, Bensen, & White, 1969). The choice of surgery depends upon the nature of the failure to obtain a good oronasal seal (Bumsted, 1982).

Speech assessment, including audiometry and speech therapy, are usual before secondary surgery to determine the degree of speech impairment and the possibility of improvement with speech rehabilitation attempts. In some cases of minor nasal escape, speech therapy alone may bring about sufficiently normal speech. When this is not possible, surgery will, it is hoped, produce better function of the sphincter mechanism. However, exercises to improve nasopharyngeal closure in speech may be necessary after surgery. The correction of cleft palate consonant substitutions (e.g., glottal stops for plosives and nasopharyngeal fricatives for sibilants and affricates) will require much time and patience in order to break the patterns of years of habit (M. Edwards, 1980).

## Deep Pharynx/Short Palate

A congenital defect in which there is insufficient closure of the palatopharyngeal sphincter may occur. The soft palate may appear to be short or the pharynx too deep and wide. The condition may be revealed only after adenoidectomy. A course of speech therapy to correct excessive nasality should be followed. If speech does not improve, a full investigative procedure should be followed, as for cleft palate, and a palatal push-back and pharyngoplasty considered.

## Laryngeal Abnormalities

Congenital abnormalities of the larynx are relatively rare, but all cases of hoarseness and of pitch irregularities should be investigated in children laryngoscopically. Laryngeal anomalies include disparity in size and level of the vocal cords, arytenoid fixation, or agenesis. Membranous webs across the anterior portion of the folds are found. In boys the anomaly may not be detected until puberty when the voice fails to break, and in girls the voice may remain conspicuously high and thin and fail to mature. Voice therapy is of little use in these cases, and surgical intervention is difficult and often considered inadvisable (Luchsinger & Arnold, 1965).

Acquired laryngeal abnormalities are those following gunshot wounds, injuries from flying glass, or blows suffered in car crashes (Looper & Figi, 1976). The thyroid cartilage may be fractured and the vocal cords displaced and torn. Holinger, Schild, and Maurizi (1968) advocate early repair as soon as the patient is well enough in order to avoid healing and stenosis while the tracheotomy tube is present. There is then a good prognosis for the voice, although the eventual result will depend largely upon the condition of the laryngeal muscles and normality of movement. Speech therapy may improve the voice and should be tried.

# Neurological Disorders

## Paralysis of the Palate

Congenital paralysis of the palate is a rare cause of excessive nasality in speech. It may only be detected after adenoidectomy when the pad of adenoids, which has made palatopharyngeal closure possible, is removed. Correction of impaired palatal function is difficult. A pharyngoplasty operation is not very successful (Wynn-Williams, 1958). A palatal prosthesis may be the best remedy. Paralysis of the palate may not be the only sign of neurological damage and occurs in cerebral palsy.

Paralysis of the palate is more frequently an acquired condition. Diptheria used to be a common cause of temporary neural paralysis, but immunization has made the disease a rarity. Poliomyelitis can also paralyze the palate, but movement may improve and speech therapy is helpful. Again immunization has eradicated the disease in the Western world but not in the Third World.

## Laryngeal Palsy

Congenital paralysis of the vocal cords will probably be detected at birth on account of breathing difficulties. A unilateral paralysis may not be diagnosed until hoarseness, vocal weakness, or inability to sing leads to a laryngoscopy examination later in life. Endotracheal intubation can cause paralysis, especially in premature infants, and is an increasing problem (Papsidero & Pashley, 1980). It is also a cause of vocal cord paralysis in long-lasting laryngeal obstruction following laryngeal trauma. The need to perform a tracheostomy early in such patients is not always recognized. When only one cord is affected, the healthy cord can pass over the midline to meet the other, and little vocal impairment results.

Pressure on the recurrent laryngeal nerves can cause paresis of the laryngeal muscles and a weak (aesthenic) voice. The vocal change can be the first sign of disease—which is why, as emphasized earlier, careful investigation and diagnosis are essential. It is all too easy to attribute ill-defined complaints of tiredness of the throat and voice to imagination and nerves. There are many possibilities of early organic and systemic disease. These are pressure from tumors in the neck and apices of the lungs, enlarged thyroid gland, aortic aneurysm, and mitral stenosis. Neurological diseases such as myasthenia gravis and Parkinson's disease can occur.

Thyroidectomy, the partial or total removal of the thyroid gland due to overfunctioning of the gland or neoplasm, is the most common cause of laryngeal palsy on account of the gland's position in close relation to the laryngeal nerves. Both recurrent and superior laryngeal nerves are at risk at operation. Riddell (1970) reported the very low incidence of 0.6% damage when the nerves were identified and 2% when visualization during operation proved impossible.

De Souza (1980) states that the nerves should be identified and preserved. Improved surgical techniques during the preceding decade make damage unlikely except in the case of diffuse tumor.

If damage to the recurrent laryngeal nerves occurs, the degree of voice impairment depends upon the resulting position of the cords (see Figure 7). A unilateral paralysis with the cord in the paramedian or intermediate position

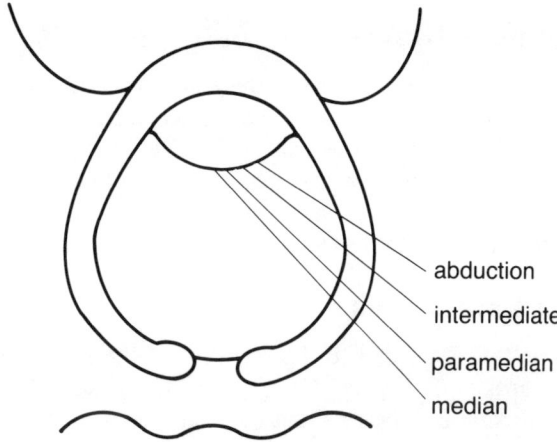

**Figure 7.** Vocal cord positions in palsies.

results generally in immediate postoperative aphonia with gradual recovery of a hoarse voice. Speech therapy in these cases can result in improvement. The affected vocal cord may recover movement altogether or in the course of time gradually move nearer the midline, while the healthy cord may compensate and swing over the midline to meet the opposite cord. Increase in volume of phonic air must be developed, and vocal exercises with hard attack must be practiced at frequent intervals during the day for short periods. Forceful exercises, such as pushing against a table, or pushing down on a chair and lifting the body while phonating, stimulate sphincteric closure of the glottis on effort. Such exercises can produce laryngitis and strain and should be practiced in moderation.

If the voice does not recover adequately and remains weak after a period of 6 months because the affected cord is in the intermediate or paramedian position, excellent vocal recovery can be achieved by injecting Teflon into the affected cord. The voice recovers immediately and dramatically in most cases (Von Leden, Yanagihara, & Werner-Kukuk, 1967).

Isshiki (1980) describes the extreme delicacy of the cordal injection operation. The exact site and the amount of Teflon injected are crucial since the result is irreversible. The mucosal elasticity of the vocal mucous membrane must be preserved. Overinjection of Teflon can render the cord bulky and stiff so that it cannot vibrate adequately. The procedure is most successful in the treatment of unilateral vocal cord paralysis and should not be attempted in the remedy of dysphonia due to atrophy, trauma, corrugated vocal edges, or radiation therapy.

## Myasthenia Gravis

Myasthenia gravis is a failure of the body to produce acetyl choline, which is necessary for the conduction of the motor impulse from nerve end plates to muscle. This produces weakness in all movements, which increases with activity. Weakness of the voice and nasality may be the first early signs of disease. The patient is treated with neostigmine or given a thymectomy. Speech therapy is not prescribed once the vocal deterioration is correctly diagnosed.

## Parkinson's Disease

Parkinson's disease, due to degeneration of the basal ganglia, exhibits symptoms of spastic rigidity and tremor, also dyskinesia. The onset of the disease may be unilateral or bilateral but eventually involves both sides of the body. It is a curious aspect of the disease that speech and voice are not always impaired, and symptoms can vary greatly with individual sufferers. The voice may become weak and speech slightly dysarthric as the first symptoms of the illness appear, but in advanced disease a patient's speech disturbance can be minimal. At worst, speech is unintelligible and very rapid, the voice is weak and tremulous, rhythm and stress are lost, and articulatory movements trail off into an incoherent mumble.

This festination of speech is due to an increase in the speed of movement and a decrease in the range of movements. All bodily movements, not only those of the speech mechanism, are affected. Walking is difficult, and writing exhibits tremor and diminishing size. All movement can suddenly come to a standstill, and initiation of movement can be difficult. A typical cog-wheel movement is diagnostic on manipulation of the elbow joint or wrist. A head tremor is often an early sign. The facial expression becomes masklike, giving a misleading impression of unfriendliness.

The actual etiology of Parkinson's disease is the failure of the substantia nigra in the corpus callosum to excrete dopamine. Treatment used to be confined to stereotactic thalamomy (Selby, 1967). Since the manufacture of the dopaminergic drug L-dopa, surgical procedures are largely abandoned, but resource to thalamotomy may be considered for patients who cannot tolerate the drugs. Dopamine therapy produces good results for periods of 7 to 10 years, but eventually the sufferer deteriorates both mentally and physically.

The effects of neurochemotherapy on patients with impaired speech have proved disappointing. Reports are conflicting, probably due to the speech parameters assessed and variation in drug dosages. Logemann, Fisher, Boshes, and Blonsky (1978) found 80% of 200 patients had altered phonation but did not find that speech improved with L-dopa. Wolfe, Garvin, Bacon, and Waldrop (1975) rated the four parameters voice, articulation, pitch variation, and rate of utterance before and after drug therapy. They found that the first three improved, but the rate of speech did not.

The results of speech therapy are disappointing, which explains the fact that not many Parkinson's disease patients are referred for speech therapy. They are cared for by physiotherapists and occupational therapists who help to keep patients mobile and self-sufficient in their homes for as long as possible.

Patients respond to procedures to slow down speech and improve articulation, volume, and inflection in a clinical setting but find it impossible to transfer this improved control to conversation. The chief cause of the trouble has always been recognized as impairment of proprioceptive impulses involving muscles, tendons, and joints. However, treatment using biofeedback and visual displays indicates that these patients also fail to monitor speech by ear. This became evident when given auditory and visual biofeedback training. Patients with Parkinson's disease required instruction and much practice before they could recognize vocal faults and correct them through auditory and visual channels. Greene and Watson (1968) found some patients benefitted considerably from use of a pocket speech amplifier, asserting that they could then hear themselves better. Scott and Caird (1983) used a Vocalite lamp, which responds to volume and duration of sound so that vocal volume, rate, and rhythm of speech can be monitored. An hour's treatment per day for 2 weeks was given, and the improvement gained was maintained for the follow-up period of 6 months. Downie, Low, and Lindsay (1981), experimenting with delayed auditory feedback, found that 2 patients out of a group of 11 improved their festinating speech while using a DAF machine but failed to transfer this improvement into ordinary speech without it. However, wearing portable DAF instruments, the patients were able to maintain an improved standard of intelligibility.

## Cerebral Palsy

Damage to the nervous system before, during, or after birth—which is the nature of cerebral palsy—is known commonly by the term *spastic*. Neurological damage, however, is unselective; lesions can involve any part of the central nervous system and in varying combinations and degrees of muscular paralysis. A child may have symptoms of spasticity, flaccidity, athetosis, or ataxia. Intelligence, hearing, and vision can be impaired. Besides the difficulty with articulation (dysarthria) there will be dysphonia with involvement of laryngeal and respiratory muscles. The two combine in what is sometimes called *dysarthrophonia*. Speech and language delay can be expected, and the possibility of hearing loss must be kept in mind.

A pediatric neurologist is required in diagnosis and assessment. Physiotherapists play a very important role in training posture and movement. Speech therapists should collaborate early because sucking, swallowing, and breathing require help, and the specialized knowledge of a speech therapist regarding the speech musculature is important, especially as cooing and babbling develop in the baby.

Necessary to the problems of habilitation of the cerebral palsied child is a team approach involving physiotherapists, speech and occupational therapists, educational psychologists and teachers, social workers, and health visitors. These should work together to provide the best program possible for the child as well as the ongoing support needed by the parents of a severely handicapped child.

Physiotherapists and speech therapists share so many common skills in eliciting improvement in motor control that they must work together closely, especially with the problems of breathing and the posture of the trunk, head, and neck, commencing with showing the mother how best to manage feeding the baby. Cerebral palsy has developed as a speciality within speech pathology because remedial methods are largely based upon neurological knowledge (Luchsinger & Arnold, 1965). For example, speech treatment for spastic dysarthrophonia may rely upon reflex inhibition, which is the basis of the Bobath method. Abnormal reflex activity is inhibited and normal automatic reactions facilitated. Within the neurophysiologic framework the speech therapist can introduce and adapt the fundamental principles of voice and speech production. Icing and brushing the lips, tongue, and facial muscles; manipulation by pressure, stretch, and resistance in the muscles of articulation; and tapping and vibration may all be used. These strategies employed by physiotherapists are known as proprioceptive neuromuscular facilitation (PNF) (Eldred, 1967; Hollis, 1976; Knott & Voss, 1968; Mysak, 1963).

Habilitation depends largely on the degree of damage to the nervous system. Intelligence, hearing, emotional stability, motivation, and parental support can achieve remarkable progress in some of the most severe cases. Maturation of the nervous system often leads to unexpected improvement in motor control, enabling the child to become mobile and lead a reasonably normal life.

## Suprabulbar Palsy (Pseudobulbar Palsy)

Patients suffering from arteriosclerosis, especially over the age of 65, are prone to diffuse cerebral vascular accidents. Bilateral lesions in the fronto-bulbar tracts cause spastic paralysis of oral, pharyngeal, and laryngeal muscles. Swallowing is difficult, and drooling occurs. Speech is badly affected, articulation slurred and slow, the voice drawling and nasalized, and pitch low and monotonous. Phrases are reduced to a few words at a time, and the muscles tire quickly. Reflex movements of chewing and swallowing are less impaired than voluntary speech movements.

Besides a speech assessment, the geriatric patient's needs regarding eyesight, hearing, and dentures must not be forgotten. The dentures may no longer fit, and an orthodontist should be consulted since an unstable denture renders articulation that much more difficult. If there is a facial palsy, ulceration of the inside cheek can be caused by repeated biting on slack muscle. Selley (1977) recommends building a shelf on a denture above the gum to protect the cheek from chewing movements. Drooling of saliva is distressing to the patient, and Tudor and Selley (1974) have used a palatal training device that incorporates biofeedback training and has been found useful with dysarthric patients in supervised therapy sessions. Speech therapy can help the dysarthric patient make the best use of what movement remains and give encouragement to persevere in attempts to speak. The palsy is progressive since further vascular accidents are to be expected. As long as the patient remains mentally alert, communication by writing is possible and electronic aids can be used, such as the Canon Communicator, which is virtually a minitypewriter strapped to the wrist.

Electronic speaking aids are now being made that will be a boon to those who cannot produce intelligible speech. Battery-operated and portable speaking instruments are already available. For example, the CONVAID, which has a voice module and a keyboard, provides unlimited possibilities for storing words and phrases. The elements stored in the machine's memory are released as speech by pressing a key. Such machines are still in their infancy but hold great promise for the future.

# Tumors of the Larynx

## Papilloma (Papillomata)

Papilloma of the larynx are benign epithelial tumors that do not invade muscular tissue and are primarily a childhood complaint. Juvenile papilloma of the larynx is a serious and distressing condition on account of the interference in breathing. The child must be kept constantly under supervision because the growths may proliferate suddenly. The cause is now considered to be a virus infection and not a hormonal problem, as was once considered to be the case, because papilloma disappear during puberty and recur in later life.

The most effective and generally practiced form of treatment is plucking the papilloma off the mucous membrane with forceps. This, with microsurgical techniques, should cause no damage to the vocal cords. In very small children a tracheostomy with valve cannula or "speaking tube" may be preferable.

Brondbo, Alberti, and Crowson (1983) regard forceps removal as hazardous and advocate vaporizing by laser in adult cases. This is not a cure but prolongs remission (Sorenson, 1982).

The voice of the child will be breathy, hoarse, or aphonic according to the degree of laryngeal obstruction caused by the papillomata. After surgical or laser removal, and especially after recurrence in the adult and periods of inability to adduct the cords, tension and upper thoracic breathing have generally become firmly established. Voice therapy will be beneficial. Increase in volume of phonic respiration and practice of prolonged phonation of vowels form the basis of treatment.

Wilson (1979) describes successful speech therapy after dispersal of papilloma, but there is some disagreement among experts concerning the benefit and indeed advisability of voice therapy. Boone (1977) states that speech therapy should not be given under any circumstances while papilloma are present. Cooper (1971) holds the contrary view and believes that voice therapy can reduce and even eliminate the growths. Greene (1980) remarks that since papilloma resemble warts—which, as everyone knows, can be spirited away by magic, suggestion, and strange rituals—speech therapy may well act like magic. In any case, a child who attempts to make his or her hoarse voice heard will subject the larynx to much strain and must suffer from vocal abuse. This may damage the delicate mucous membrane cover of the vocal cords and encourage the spread of infection.

### Cancer of the Larynx

The first sign of cancer developing in the vocal cords is hoarseness—hence the vital necessity to consult a laryngologist if sudden hoarseness persists for more than 4 weeks. Cancer of the larynx is rare under 40 years but can occur in adolescence. Tumors limited to the vocal cords are curable by irradiation because lymphatic drainage is negligible and metastasis unlikely. The throat is uncomfortably dry and the voice hoarse during and after radiotherapy, but this ameliorates and speech therapy is not necessary. A chronic laryngitis may persist after irradiation or reappear in patients who use their voices considerably, in which case speech therapy can help, but frequently the laryngitis is due to a recurrence of the malignancy.

# Laryngectomy and Esophageal Speech

In Britain the conventional and conservative approach to a recurrence of cordal carcinoma is total laryngectomy, so that patients referred for speech therapy after laryngofissure (partial laryngectomy) are few. There is, however, no reason why a laryngofissure, or some other method of subtotal laryngectomy, should not be done if only a stage one carcinoma is present (Sessions, Maness, & McSwain, 1965; Shaw, 1966).

The operation of laryngofissure is far less traumatic than that of total laryngectomy since a normal airway and a normal laryngeal voice, though hoarse, are preserved. For this reason in the United States subtotal or partial laryngectomy is frequently preferred to total laryngectomy. Recently gained knowledge relating the anatomy of the larynx to the spread of cancer and its escape routes via the submucosal lymphatic compartments has brought about changes in surgery. The significance of superficial and deep lymph routes and the embryological development of the larynx in two halves is recognized. Whereas a superficial tumor in the mucosa of the larynx may travel freely across the midline of the larynx and invade the other side, the deeper structures do not readily communicate from one side to the other (Pressman & Bailey, 1968). Various vertical, horizontal, and frontolateral procedures are carried out (Kirchener, 1978). American surgeons have developed great skill in carrying out operations for partial removal of the larynx in very early cancer, sparing the patient's voice and respiratory airway (Berry, 1983). Hemilaryngectomy, anterior commisure resection, and supraglottic procedures have proved to be more successful in eradicating disease (Ogura & Thawley, 1977). Total laryngectomy is held in reserve for those cases where conservation surgery can no longer control cancer invasion.

Removal of the larynx, which is necessary when radiotherapy and conservation surgery have failed, is a traumatic experience, leaving the patient and his or her family shocked and anxious. Apart from the fear of cancer recurrence, the patient has to contend with loss of voice coupled with the distressing change in the respiratory tract. The trachea, severed below the larynx, is sutured to a stoma at the base of the neck through which breathing and coughing take place (see Figure 8). A severe depression may set in that is detrimental to the recovery and adaptation of the laryngectomee (Darvill, 1983; Heaver & Arnold, 1962). With adequate support and counselling the patient and family can be helped through the early days and weeks before and after the operation (Murrills, 1983).

The whole team concerned with the work of rehabilitation may consist of surgeon, radiotherapist, nurses, doctors, physiotherapist and speech pathologist, social workers, and successfully rehabilitated laryngectomees (Glover, 1983). Careful explanation of every step, both before and after surgery, needs to be understood. Since loss of voice will be the worst problem to face, the speech pathologist plays an all-important role before and after the operation. The patient needs to talk to laryngectomees before the operation and ask ques-

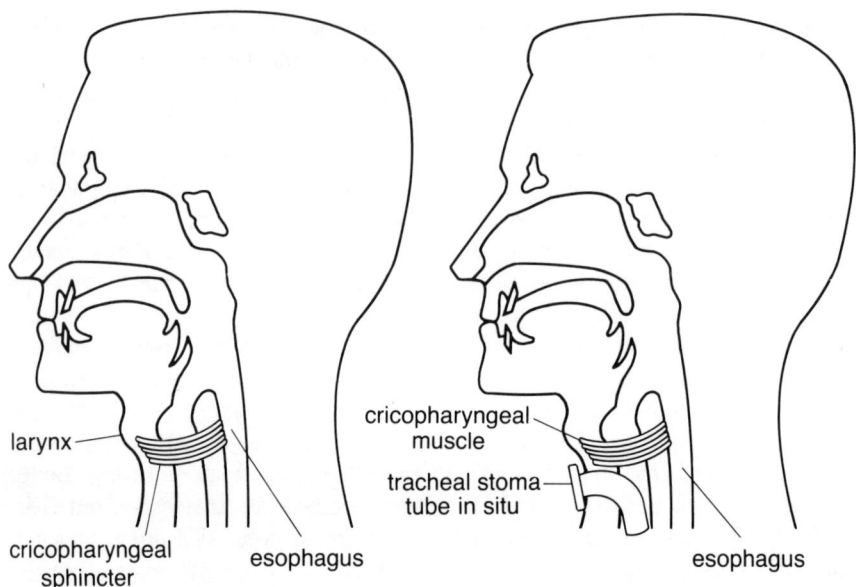

**Figure 8.** Before and after laryngectomy.

tions of somebody who has come through the experience and is leading a normal life. A Cooper-Rand oral reed vibrator can be used immediately after the operation, which means there is no need for the patient to write things down or to strain the unhealed wound in an attempt to whisper. The patient should practice with the instrument before the laryngectomy so that it can be used without worry and fatigue when talking to nurses, doctors, and visitors after laryngectomy.

It will probably be several months before the laryngectomee is proficient in producing esophageal voice and encouragement should be given to transfer to a throat-placed vibrator once the condition of the throat allows. The patient should also have access to a number of different electronic larynges, as personal preferences and the type most suitable to the particular throat resonance vary. The most expensive type — with volume and pitch controls — may not necessarily be the best for a particular individual. Use of a vibrator while attending voice therapy sessions to develop esophageal voice allows instant communication with family and friends, use of a telephone, and early return to work and a normal life, which might otherwise be delayed. There are differing estimates of the percentage of laryngectomees who do not develop adequate esophageal speech, but all of them are disappointingly high. Edwards (1976) estimated that at least 30% fail. Goode (1975) put failure rates as high as 50%. As radiotherapy and early surgical intervention lead to more cures, the laryngectomy operations with esophageal and pharyngeal extensions (Loré, 1978) naturally inflate the numbers failing to speak. At best, esophageal speech is never loud, so a speaker finds it very tiring to speak for lengthy periods and against background noise. Perry (1983a) states that normal laryngeal voice is produced at 65–70 dB, rising to 95 dB, whereas the average level esophageal voice is 40–50 dB. When speech is fluent but lacking volume, a pocket amplifier with hand-held microphone, throat microphone, or headset with speaking tube can help the speaker (Greene, 1980). Telephones can also be fitted with an amplification unit which makes things easier, but generally esophageal voice can be understood clearly over the phone.

In a simple laryngectomy operation the cricopharyngeal muscle is carefully detached from the cricoid cartilage, leaving intact the cricopharyngeal sphincter, which encircles the top of the esophagus. This muscle forms the vibrator for esophageal voice and is activated by expulsion of air from the esophagus. A few cubic centimeters of esophageal air is enough to produce a vowel. Since the cricopharyngeal muscle is composed of striated muscle innervated by the recurrent laryngeal nerve, a laryngectomee can acquire the knack of relaxation during air charge and tensing on expulsion of air so that the muscle folds vibrate or cause air turbulence. Control of pseudovoice develops to a remarkable degree in many patients, and a good speaker can produce acceptable tone, volume, inflection, and phrasing. Speech may be of such excellence that a stranger may think that the patient's hoarse voice is due to a cold, but such excellence is rare.

There are various ways in which the esophagus may be charged with air. First, it can be swallowed, but this is unsuitable except as a means of letting the patient get the feel of what is wanted. The air tends to travel down into the stomach and cannot be controlled, causing discomfort. Fizzy drinks can also be used, since burping up the gas can give the sound and feel of esophageal voice in early stages.

Second, a glossopharyngeal press can be used. This requires using the back of the tongue to push a bubble of air back into the pharynx. The lips need to be closed, the tongue body pressed against the hard palate, and the soft palate elevated in a sort of munching movement.

Another means of injecting air into the esophagus is to pronounce plosive syllables and affricates in an exaggerated fashion.

Inhalation, or aspiration of air, is advocated as the best method of charging the "vicarious lung" by many (Diedrich & Youngstrom, 1966; Snidecor, 1968). A quick intake of air with a rapid descent of the diaphragm sucks air into the esophagus and is then expressed on vowel sounds. To achieve this, the pseudoglottis must be relaxed and not restricted by scar tissue.

Fluent speakers rely upon all methods, pressing back air from the oral cavity before speaking, inhaling, and recharging the esophagus by articulatory movements as they speak. In the early stages speech therapy must be adaptable and versatile and allow the patient to experiment and use whatever method most easily produces esophageal voice. An amplifier may help the laryngectomee to hear his or her new voice, and a vibrator can assist, not hinder, development of esophageal voice (Gardner, 1971; Lauder, 1968). The injection of air from plosive consonants is promoted by encouraging the patient to relax, breathe normally, and not force air from the stoma while uttering words which begin and end with plosives. Initial consonants /m/, /n/, /w/, /l/, and vowels should be avoided; /k/ and /g/ are best to start with since they most easily succeed in pushing an air "bubble" back into the throat.

Success in using esophageal voice depends upon many factors, the first of which is not necessarily the site and flexibility of the pseudoglottis. Age, general health, and fitness are obviously positive advantages in addition to good hearing. Motivation and encouragement from relatives and associates are essential. Some laryngectomees, especially women, prefer an artificial larynx to esophageal voice, and sometimes the spouse cannot stand the belching quality of the voice and discourages it in the partner. Individual preferences among laryngectomees and their families must be respected.

## Surgical Speech Restoration (Fistula Voice)

The high rate of failure in the acquisition of fluent esophageal speech, the difficulties and time involved, and the poor performance in aesthetic terms of the electrolarynx are all factors causing dissatisfaction and the search for alternative solutions. Surgeons have endeavored to construct in the throat of laryngectomees, at the time of the operation or later, a vibrator of living tissue that can be activated by lung air. This development is known as *fistula voice*. The advantages of such surgical techniques are very great. Lung air can be used instead of having to learn a totally new means of shunting air using the esophagus as a vicarious lung. Fistula voice needs little learning and is immediate, fluent, loud, and effortless. It is of a more acceptable tone than that of esophageal voice and a great improvement on the robot quality of electronic voice. However, the difficulties in achieving successful results are also very great. The two main problems are difficulties in healing after radiotherapy and the danger of leakage of saliva from the fistula into the trachea and down to the lungs, causing chest

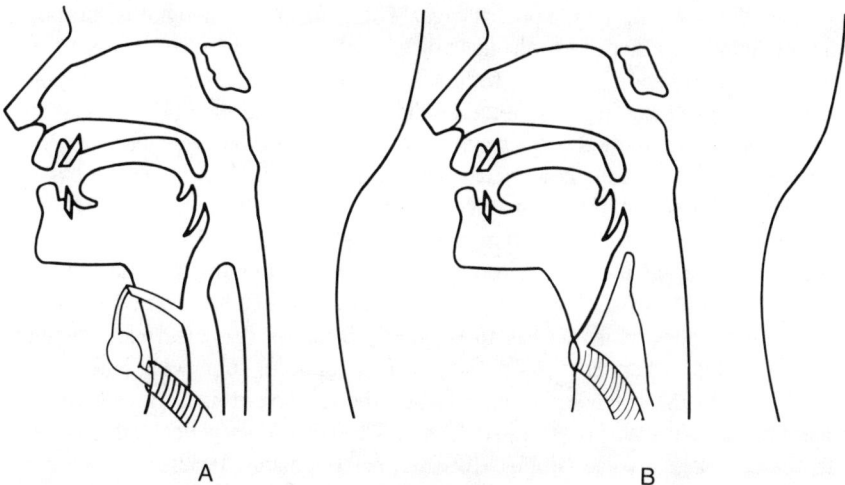

**Figure 9.** Surgical speech rehabilitation techniques. A, fistula for external prosthesis; B, Asai skin tube construction.

infection. Edwards (1976, 1983) has traced the historical evolution of surgical speech rehabilitation (SSR) in two valuable reports that are illustrated by clear diagrams.

## External Prosthesis

A vocal prosthesis worn externally is connected to the tracheostoma by a silicone tube to pick up lung air and another tube above, which is inserted into a stoma beneath the chin. This stoma is the opening of a skin tube constructed some time after laryngectomy (see Figure 9). It leads from the neck stoma into the pharynx and channels the vibrated air into the throat. Taub (1975) with his Voice Bak, Edwards (1976), and others experimented with these prostheses, which are now obsolete since the invention of internal surgical reconstruction techniques.

## Tracheal Pharyngeal Tube Construction

Asai, at the eighth ORL International Congress in 1965, described a new technique whereby he constructed a skin tube leading from the truncated trachea up to the base of the tongue with a fistula into the hypopharynx (see Figure 9). A finger placed over the tracheal stoma drives air up the speaking tube into the pharynx for speech. The hypopharyngeal fistula forms the neoglottis, producing a voice similar to that of esophageal voice. This procedure necessitates a three-stage operation and requires careful selection of patients. Asai (1972) reported good speech results in 72 patients, as did Arslan and Serafini (1972). The innovators of a new method are always more successful than their disciples, however, and the search for new techniques continued. The Asai technique has now been supplanted by the phonatory neoglottis of Staffieri (1980). This is an ingenious primary reconstruction done at the same time as laryngectomy. A tracheoesophageal tube is made out of a mucous membrane flap salvaged from the back of the larynx. The tube leads from the trachea into the esophagus.

The esophageal fistula has to be ideally 5 mm in diameter and sufficiently elastic to close when air is not passing through in order to prevent leakage from the tube into the trachea. A finger closes the trachea stoma, as with the Asai method, to direct air into the esophagus. The voice thus generated is superior to the esophageal voice (Robbins, Fisher, & Logemann, 1982).

## Tracheoesophageal Voice Valves

The Staffieri procedure has in turn been superceded by development in the past 5 years of internally sited valvular prostheses, which do not involve the difficult and delicate surgical techniques required for skin tube construction. The Blom-Singer voice button was first described by Singer and Blom (1980) and followed by a further report on a larger corpus of patients (Singer & Blom, 1983).

The Blom-Singer method does not require the construction of an epithelial-lined tube. A puncture is made simply through the trachea into the esophagus, into which is inserted a "duck-billed" valved voice prosthesis with external retention flange (see Figure 10). The valve only opens for passage of air (again under digital control) and closes to form a tight seal at all times. The prosthesis is not a vibrator but provides the passage of lung air into the esophagus at the pharyngoesophageal (cricopharyngeal) junction (Perry, 1983b). This creates esophageal voice in the usual way and is of similar quality.

The tracheoesophageal puncture closes and heals rapidly if the valve is removed, which means the valve must be worn continuously except when removed to be cleaned. The valve deteriorates after a time, and leakage causes coughing and discomfort. It must be replaced without delay. Some patients fail to produce phonation on account of constriction of the cricopharyngeal junction. Before fitting the Blom-Singer valve, an air insufflation test is advisable. Failure to acquire esophageal voice may also be a sign of overtight pharyngeal muscles.

Singer and Blom (1980) report excellent results with their Blom-Singer valve: 114 patients out of a series of 129 successfully produced voice. However, they feel that the need for manual closure is inconvenient, unhygienic, and

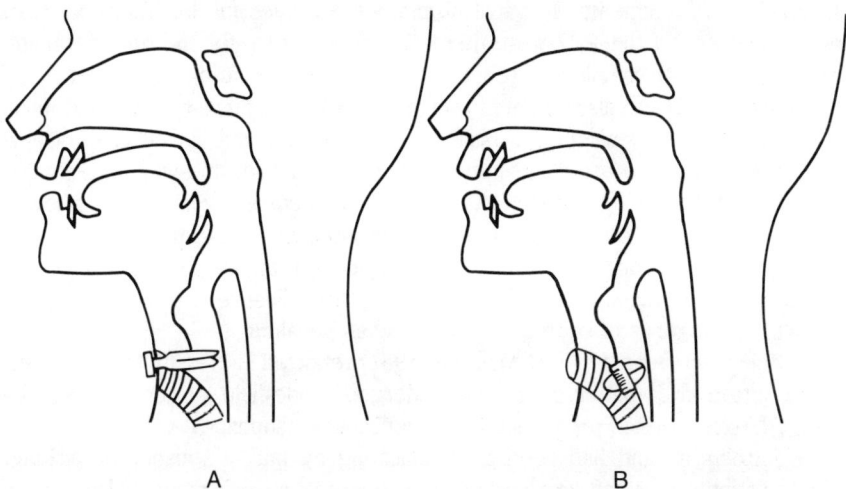

**Figure 10.** Voice buttons. A, Blom-Singer; B, Panjé.

draws attention to the disability. Recently they have designed a "breathing button" containing a sensitive diaphragm that makes direction of air through the duck-billed valve possible without recourse to using a finger. The two-way respiratory valve is fitted into the tracheal stoma. It converts to a one-way inspiratory valve with increased breath pressure for voice and thus replaces digital closure to direct air into the esophagus via the duck-billed valve. When the wearer is exercising or coughing, the valve adjusts and the diaphragm automatically inverts and everts with increased inspiration and expiration.

Singer and Blom (1980) stress the need for surgeon and speech therapist to work together throughout management of the patient with voice valve prosthesis. The speech pathologist assists in the selection of the right length of prosthetic tube suitable for each patient and also teaches the patient how to remove and clean the valve daily and replace it. Relaxation, reassurance, and encouragement will be necessary, and breath control for voicing and articulation instruction may be needed.

Donegan, Gluckman, and Singh (1981) have drawn attention to the limitations of the Blom-Singer valve. They acknowledge fully the dramatic advance in neoglottic reconstruction it represents but emphasize that Blom and Singer's success ratings are misleading. Most patients fitted with the valve prosthesis can produce voice, but the real criterion for success is whether the patient is willing and able to retain the prosthesis. Donegan, Gluckman, and Singh (1981) found that of 20 patients, 13 valve fittings were successful, but there were 10 actual failures. Of these, 7 were due to inability to care for the prosthesis and the other 3 to an inability to produce fluent speech wearing the valve.

Panjé (1981) has also invented prosthesis that is of simpler design and more easily inserted. It consists of a biflanged silicone tube and valve. The tracheal end is open, and the esophageal end contains a four-flap, one-way flutter valve (see Figure 10). A puncture is made in the tracheosophageal wall at a lower level than for the Blom-Singer, and the prosthesis is inserted using a wire inserter. A flange on the tracheal side and another on the esophageal side of the tracheopharyngeal wall hold the valve in place. Closure of the tracheal neck stoma by a finger is of course necessary when speaking.

Panjé, Van Denmark, and McCabe (1981) reported successful fitting of their voice button in 24 patients who had undergone wide-field surgery and irradiation. All except 3 had previously failed to produce esophageal voice and to use an electrolarynx and had been communicating by buccal whisper or writing. Three patients who had previously used esophageal speech requested the Panjé prosthesis because their voices were weak and not sustained. The Panjé vocal rehabilitation procedure is referred to by the authors incidentally as "the stab technique for tracheoesophageal (TE) fistula."

Fistula speech with and without voice prosthesis is in the early stages of development. Each technique has its advantages and disadvantages. The traditional use of esophageal voice and/or electrolarynx will still be the preference of many patients, depending on age, health, prognosis, and personal choice. The role of the speech pathologist in rehabilitation is still a vital one and is not diminished by SSR but rather enhanced. This is a highly specialized field in which the therapist collaborates as a consultant with the surgeon and is responsible for management of the patient before and after the fitting of the valve prosthesis or skin tube reconstruction.

Speech rehabilitation has assumed a new dimension with SSR techniques. The next step may be toward the invention of a miniature electronic vibrator contained in a voice button in place of an air valve. Remote control of the device should not be beyond the bounds of human ingenuity and invention. The advantage would be the simulation of a voice more acceptable than esophageal speech, which, despite recent innovations, still remains a travesty of personal identity.

# References

Abberton, E., & Fourcin, A. (1972). Laryngographic analysis and intonation. *British Journal of Disorders of Communication, 7,* 24–29.

Amerman, J., & Williams, D. (1979). Implication of respirometric evaluation for diagnosis and management of vocal fold pathologies. *British Journal of Disorders of Communication, 14,* 153–160.

Arnold, G., & Heaver, L. (1959). Spastic dysphonia. *Logos, 2,* 3–24.

Aronson, A. (1973). *Audio-seminar in psychogenic voice disorders.* Philadelphia: Saunders.

Aronson, A. (1980). *Clinical voice disorders.* New York: Thieme-Stratton.

Aronson, A., Brown, J., Litin, E., & Pearson, J. (1968a). Spastic dysphonia: I. Voice, neurologic, and psychiatric aspects. *Journal of Speech and Hearing Disorders, 33,* 203–218.

Aronson, A., Brown, J., Litin, E., & Pearson, J. (1968b). Spastic dysphonia: II. Comparison with essential (voice) tremor and other neurologic and psychogenic dysphonias. *Journal of Speech and Hearing Disorders, 33,* 219–231.

Arslan, M., & Serafini, I. (1972). Restoration of laryngeal functions after total laryngectomy: Report on the first 25 cases. *Laryngoscope, 82,* 1349–1360.

Asai, R. (1972). Laryngoplasty after total laryngectomy. *Archives of Otolaryngology, 95,* 114–119.

Bass, C., & Gardner, W. (1984). The hyperventilation syndrome. *Cardiology in Practice, 2,* 26–34.

Beckett, R. (1971). A respirometer as a diagnostic and clinical tool in the speech clinic. *Journal of Speech and Hearing Disorders, 36,* 235–241.

Bernstein, L. (1979). Cleft lip and palate. In G. English (Ed.), *Otolaryngology* (Vol. 4, Chap. 18, pp. 1–39). New York: Harper & Row.

Berry, R., Epstein, R., Fourcin, A., Freeman, M., MacCurtain, F., & Noscoe, N. (1982). An objective analysis of voice disorders, I and II. *British Journal of Disorders of Communication, 17,* 67–83.

Berry, R. (1983). Radiotherapy and chemotherapy. In Y. Edels (Ed.), *Laryngectomy: Diagnosis to rehabilitation* (pp. 18–35). Beckenham, England: Croom Helm.

Boone, D. (1977). *The voice and voice therapy.* Englewood Cliffs, NJ: Prentice-Hall.

Bowden, R. (1974). Innervation of intrinsic laryngeal muscles. In B. Wyke (Ed.), *Ventilatory and phonatory control systems* (pp. 370–382). London: Oxford University Press.

Brodnitz, F. (1971). *Vocal rehabilitation.* Rochester, MN: Whiting Press.

Brøndbo, K., Alberti, P., & Crowson, N. (1983). Adult recurrent multiple laryngeal papilloma: Laser management and socio-economic effects. *Acta Oto-Laryngologica, 95,* 431–439.

Bumsted, R. (1982). Velopharyngeal incompetence. In G. English (Ed.), *Otolaryngology* (Vol. 4, Chap. 40, pp. 1–25). New York: Harper & Row.

Campbell, E., Agostini, E., & Newsom-Davis, J. (1970). *The respiratory muscles: Mechanics and neural control.* London: Lloyd-Luke Medical Books.

Campbell, E. (1974). Muscular activity in normal and abnormal ventilation. In B. Wyke (Ed.), *Ventilatory and phonatory control systems* (pp. 3–11). London: Oxford University Press.

Cooper, M. (1971). Papillomata of the vocal folds—a review. *Journal of Speech and Hearing Disorders, 36,* 51–60.

Cooper, M. (1973). *Modern techniques of vocal rehabilitation.* Springfield, IL: Thomas.

Cooper, M. (1974). Spectrographic analysis of fundamental frequency and hoarseness before and after vocal rehabilitation. *Journal of Speech and Hearing Disorders, 39,* 286–297.

Cooper, M., & Cooper, M. (Eds.). (1977). *Approaches to vocal rehabilitation.* Springfield, IL: Thomas.

Cooper, M., & Nahum, A. (1971). Vocal rehabilitation for contact ulcer of the larynx. *Archives of Otolaryngology, 85,* 41–46.

Dalton, P. (1983). Maintenance of change: Towards the integration of behavioural and psychological procedures. In P. Dalton (Ed.), *Approaches to the treatment of stuttering* (pp. 163–184). London: Croom Helm.

Damsté, P. (1964). Virilisation of the voice due to anabolic steroids. *Folia Phoniatrica, 16,* 10–18.

Darvill, G. (1983). Rehabilitation—not just voice. In Y. Edels (Ed.), *Laryngectomy: Diagnosis to rehabilitation* (pp. 192–217). London: Croom Helm.

Dedo, H. (1976). Recurrent laryngeal nerve section for spastic dysphonia. *Journal of Laryngology and Otology, 85,* 451–459.

Dedo, H., & Lawson, L. (1977). Recurrent laryngeal section and postoperative speech therapy for spasmodic (spastic) dysphonia. *Proceedings of the 17th International Association of Logopedics and Phoniatrics Congress* (Vol. 1, pp. 131–135). Copenhagen: International Association of Logopedics and Phoniatrics.

Dedo, H., & Shipp, T. (1980). *Spastic dysphonia—a surgical and voice treatment program.* Houston: College Hill Press.

Dedo, H., Townsend, J., & Isdebski, K. (1978). Current evidence for organic etiology in spastic dysphonia. *Journal of Laryngology and Otology, 86,* 875–880.

De Souza, F. (1980). Thyroidectomy. In G. English (Ed.), *Otolaryngology* (Vol. 5, Chap. 49, pp. 1–15). Philadelphia: Lippincott.

Diedrich, W., & Youngstrom, K. (1966). *Alaryngeal speech.* Springfield, IL: Thomas.

Donegan, J., Gluckman, J., & Singh, J., (1981). Limitations of the Blom-Singer technique for voice restoration. *Annals of Oto-Rhino-Laryngology, 90,* 495–497.

Downie, A., Low, J., & Lindsay, D. (1981). Speech disorder in Parkinsonism: Usefulness of delayed auditory feedback in selected cases. *British Journal of Disorders of Communication, 16,* 135–139.

Dunker, E., & Schlosshauer, B. (1964). Irregularities of the laryngeal vibratory patterns in healthy and hoarse persons. In D. Brewer (Ed.), *Research potential in voice physiology* (pp. 151–184). Syracuse: State University of New York, Upstate Medical Center.

Edwards, M. (1980). Assessment and remediation of speech. In M. Edwards & A. Watson (Eds.), *Cleft palate: Advances in management* (pp. 190–205). London: Churchill-Livingstone.

Edwards, N. (1976). The artificial larynx. *British Journal of Hospital Medicine, 16,* 145–164.

Edwards, N. (1983). The surgical approach to speech rehabilitation. In Y. Edels (Ed.), *Laryngectomy: Diagnosis to rehabilitation* (pp. 249–270). Beckenham, England: Croom Helm.

Eldred, E. (1967). Peripheral receptors: Their excitation and relation to reflex patterns. *American Journal of Physical Medicine, 46,* 69–87.

Fairbanks, G. (1960). *Voice and articulation drillbook.* New York: Harper.

Fourcin, A. (1981). Laryngographic assessment of phonatory function. In C. Ludlow & M. Hart (Eds.), *Proceedings of the conference on the assessment of vocal pathology* (ASHA Reports 11). Rockville, MD: American Speech and Hearing Association.

Fourcin, A., & Abberton, E. (1977). The laryngograph and the voiscope in speech therapy. *Proceedings of the 16th International Association of Logopedics and Phoniatrics Congress* (pp. 116–122). Copenhagen: International Association of Logopedics and Phoniatrics.

Fritzell, B., Feuer, E., Haglund, S., Knutsson, E., & Schiratzki, H. (1982). Experience with recurrent laryngeal nerve section for spastic dysphonia. *Folia Phoniatrica, 34,* 160–167.

Fritzell, B., Sundberg, J., & Strange-Ebbesen, A. (1982). Pitch change after stripping oedematous vocal folds. *Folia Phoniatrica, 34,* 29–32.

Froeschels, E. (1952). Chewing method as therapy: A discussion with some philosophical conclusions. *Archives of Otolaryngology, 56,* 427–434.

Gardner, W. (1971). *Laryngectomee speech and rehabilitation.* Springfield, IL: Thomas.

Gawel, M. (1981). The effects of various drugs on speech. *British Journal of Disorders of Communication, 16,* 51–57.

Glover, J. (1983). Teamwork in the care of the laryngectomee. In Y. Edels (Ed.), *Laryngectomy: Diagnosis to rehabilitation* (pp. 51–57). Beckenham, England: Croom Helm.

Goode, R. (1975). Artificial laryngeal devices in post-laryngectomy rehabilitation. *Laryngoscope, 85,* 677–689.

Gould, W. (1971). Effect of respiratory and postural mechanisms upon the action of the vocal cords. *Folia Phoniatrica, 23,* 211–224.

Gould, W., & Okamura, H. (1974). Interrelationship between voice and laryngeal mucosal reflexes. In B. Wyke (Ed.), *Ventilatory and phonatory control systems* (pp. 347–360). London: Oxford University Press.

Greene, M. (1980). *The voice and its disorders.* New York: Lippincott.

Greene, M. (1982). Aging of the voice. In M. Edwards (Ed.), *Communication changes in the elderly* (pp. 62–68). London: College of Speech Therapists.

Greene, M. (1984). Functional disphonia and the hypeventilation syndrome. *British Journal of Disorders of Communication, 19,* 263–272.

Greene, M., Timmons, B., & Glover, J. (1983). Anxiety state and the chronic hyperventilation syndrome: Relevance in speech and voice disorders. *Proceedings of the 19th International Congress of Logopedics and Phoniatrics* (pp. 704–709). London: College of Speech Therapists.

Greene, M., Timmons, B., & Glover, J. (1984). The significance of anxiety and breathing disorders in functional dysphonias. *Bulletin Européen de Physiologie Respiratoire, 20*, 94.

Greene, M., & Watson, B. (1968). The value of speech amplification in Parkinson's disease patients. *Folia Phoniatrica, 20*, 250–257.

Gross, W., & Johnson, C. (1977). Nasal fractures. In G. English (Ed.), *Otolaryngology* (Vol. 4, Chap. 26N, pp. 1–16). New York: Harper & Row.

Hardonk, J., & Beumer, M. (1979). Hyperventilation syndrome. In P. Vinker & G. Bruyn (Eds.), *Handbook of clinical neurology* (Vol. 38, pp. 309–360). New York: Elsevier-North Holland.

Härma, R., Sonninen, A., Vartiainen, E., Haveri, P., & Väisänen, A. (1975). Vocal polyps and nodules. *Folia Phoniatrica, 27*, 19–25.

Heaver, L., & Arnold, G. (1962). Rehabilitation of alaryngeal aphonia. *Post-Graduate Medicine, 32*, 11–17.

Heinemann, M. (1969). Myxodem und stimme. *Folia Phoniatrica, 21*, 55–62.

Hibbert, G. (1984). Hyperventilation as a cause of panic attacks. *British Medical Journal, 288*, 263–264.

Hixon, T., Mead, J., & Goldman, M. (1976). Dynamics of the chest wall during speech: Function of the thorax, rib cage, diaphragm, and abdomen. *Journal of Speech and Hearing Research, 19*, 297–356.

Holbrook, A., Rolnick, M., & Bailey, C. (1974). Treatment of vocal abuse disorders using a vocal intensity controller. *Journal of Speech and Hearing Disorders, 39*, 298–303.

Hollinger, P., Schild, J., & Maurizi, D. (1968). Internal and external trauma to the larynx. *Laryngoscope, 78*, 944–954.

Hollis, M. (1976). *Proprioceptive neuromuscular facilitation*. London: Blackwell.

Innocenti, D. (1983). Chronic hyperventilation syndrome. In P. Downie (Ed.), *Cash's textbook of chest, heart and vascular disorders for physiotherapists* (pp. 356–366). London: Faber & Faber.

Isshiki, N. (1964). Regulatory mechanisms of voice intensity variation. *Journal of Speech and Hearing Research, 17*, 17–29.

Isshiki, N. (1980). Recent advances in phonosurgery. *Folia Phoniatrica, 32*, 119–154.

Jackson, C., & Jackson, C. (1935). Contact ulcer of the larynx. *Archives of Otolaryngology, 22*, 1–15.

Jacobson, E. (1934). *You must relax*. New York: McGraw-Hill.

Jacobson, E. (1938). *Progressive relaxation*. Chicago: University of Chicago Press.

Jacobson, E. (1964). *Anxiety and tension control: A physiological approach*. Philadelphia: Lippincott.

Jenkins, J. (1967). Preliminary report on the treatment of multiple papillomata by ultrasound. *Journal of Laryngology and Otology, 81*, 385–390.

Julian, W., MacCurtain, F., & Noscoe, N. (1981). Anatomical factors influencing voice quality. *Journal of Physiology, 315*, 10–11.

Kelman, A., Gordon, M., Simpson, I., & Morton, F. (1975). Assessment of vocal function by airflow measurement. *Folia Phoniatrica, 27*, 250–262.

Kirchner, J. (1978). Staging in cancer of the larynx. In G. Gerald (Ed.), *Otolaryngology* (Vol. 5, Chap. 35, pp. 1–9). Philadelphia: Lippincott.

Kleinsasser, O. (1968). *Microlaryngoscopy and microsurgery* (P. Hoffman, Trans.). Philadelphia: Saunders.

Knott, M., & Voss, D. (1963). *Proprioceptive muscular facilitation*. Philadelphia: Harper & Row.

Landes, B. (1977). Management of hyperfunction. In M. Cooper & M. Cooper (Eds.), *Approaches to rehabilitation*. Springfield, IL: Thomas.

Lauder, E. (1968). The laryngectomee and the artificial larynx. *Journal of Speech and Hearing Disorders, 33*, 147–157.

Laver, J. (1980). *The phonetic description of voice quality*. Cambridge: Cambridge University Press.

Lawrence, Van L. (1979). *Spastic dysphonia: State of the art*. New York: The Voice Foundation.

Lee, R. (1983). Adjuncts to speech therapy. In P. Dalton (Ed.), *Approaches to the treatment of stuttering*. London: Croom Helm.

Lewis, B. (1959). Hyperventilation syndrome: Clinical and physiological evaluation. *California Medicine, 91*, 121–126.

Linford-Rees, W. (1967). *A short textbook of psychiatry*. London: English University Press.

Logemann, J., Fisher, H., Boshes, B., & Blonsky, E. (1978). Frequency and co-occurrence of vocal tract dysfunctions in the speech of a large sample of Parkinson patients. *Journal of Speech and Hearing Disorders, 43*, 47–57.

Looper, E., & Figi, F. (1976). Laryngeal stenosis. In G. English (Ed.), *Otolaryngology* (Vol. 4, Chap 29, pp. 1–12). Philadelphia: Harper & Row.

Lore, J., Jr., (1978). Radical surgery of the larynx and laryngopharynx. In G. English (Ed.), *Otolaryngology* (Vol. 5, Chap. 41, pp. 1–11). Philadelphia: Lippincott.

Luchsinger, R., & Arnold, G. (1965). Vocal disorders of constitutional origin. In R. Luchsinger & G. Arnold (Eds.), *Voice, speech, and language* (pp. 167–175). London: Wadsworth.

Lum, L. (1976). The syndrome of habitual chronic hyperventilation. In D. Hill (Ed.), *Modern trends in psychosomatic medicine* (Vol. 3, pp. 196–229). London: Butterworth.

Lum, L. (1981). Hyperventilation and anxiety state. *Journal of the Royal Society of Medicine, 74*, 1–4.

Mackenzie, M. (1886). *The hygiene of the vocal organs*. London: Macmillan.

Magarian, G. (1983). Hyperventilation syndrome: Infrequently recognized common experiences of anxiety and stress. *Medicine, 61*, 219–236.

Malcomson, K. (1968). Globus hystericus velopharyngis. *Journal of Laryngology and Otology, 82*, 219–230.

Mead, J., Hixon, T., & Goldman, N. (1974). Configuration of the chest wall during speech. In B. Wyke (Ed.), *Ventilatory and phonatory control systems* (pp. 58–75). London: Oxford University Press.

Mills, W. (1906). *Voice production in singing and speaking based on scientific principles.* London: Curwen.

Moses, P. (1954). *The voice of neurosis.* New York: Grune & Stratton.

Moses, P. (1960). The psychology of the castrato voice. *Folia Phoniatrica, 12,* 204–216.

Murphy, A. (1964). *Functional voice disorders.* Englewood Cliffs, NJ: Prentice-Hall.

Murrills, G. (1983). Pre- and early post-operative care of the laryngectomee and spouse. In Y. Edels (Ed.), *Laryngectomy: Diagnosis to rehabilitation* (pp. 58–74). Beckenham, England: Croom Helm.

Mysak, E. (1963). Dysarthria and oropharyngeal reflexology: A review. *Journal of Speech and Hearing Disorders, 28,* 252–260.

Mysak, E., & Hanley, T. (1959). Aging processes in speech: Pitch and duration characteristics. *Journal of Gerontology, 13,* 309–313.

Ogura, J., & Thawley, S. (1977). Conservation laryngeal surgery and radical neck dissection. In G. English (Ed.), *Otolaryngology* (Vol. 5, Chap. 36, pp. 1–41). Philadelphia: Lippincott.

Oyer, H., & Oyer, E. (1976). *Aging and communication.* Austin, TX: PRO-ED.

Panjé, W. (1981). Prosthetic rehabilitation following laryngectomy: The voice button. *Annals of Oto-Rhino-Laryngology, 90,* 116–120.

Panjé, W., Van Denmark, D., & McCabe, B. (1981). Voice button prosthesis rehabilitation of the laryngectomee. *Annals of Oto-Rhino-Laryngology, 90,* 503–505.

Papsidero, M., & Pashley, N. (1980). Acquired stenosis of the upper airway in neonates: An increasing problem. *Annals of Oto-Rhino-Laryngology, 89,* 512–514.

Peacher, G. (1961). Vocal therapy for contact ulcer – a follow-up of seventy patients. *Laryngoscope, 71,* 37–47.

Peacher, W., & Hollinger, P. (1947). Contact ulcer of the larynx: The role of vocal reeducation. *Archives of Otolaryngology, 46,* 617–623.

Perry, A. (1983a). Assessment: What, why, how, and when to measure social, physical, communication, and psychological improvement. In Y. Edels (Ed.), *Laryngectomy: Diagnosis to rehabilitation* (pp. 75–106). Beckenham, England: Croom Helm.

Perry, A. (1983b). The speech therapist's role in surgical and prosthetic approaches to speech rehabilitation. In Y. Edels (Ed.), *Laryngectomy: Diagnosis to rehabilitation* (pp. 271–288). Beckenham, England: Croom Helm.

Pigott, R. (1983). Assessment of velopharyngeal function in cleft palate: Advances in management. In Y. Edels (Ed.), *Laryngectomy: Diagnosis to rehabilitation* (pp. 206–231). Beckenham, England: Croom Helm.

Pigott, R., Bensen, J., & White, F. (1969). Nasendoscopy in the diagnosis of velopharyngeal incompetence. *Journal of Plastic and Reconstructive Surgery, 43,* 141–147.

Pressman, J., & Bailey, B. (1968). The surgery of cancer of the larynx with special reference to subtotal laryngectomy. In J. Snidecor (Ed.), *Speech rehabilitation of the laryngectomized* (2nd ed., pp. 16–49). Springfield, IL: Thomas.

Proctor, D. (1972). Breathing mechanics during phonation and singing. In B. Wyke (Ed.), *Ventilatory and phonatory control systems* (pp. 34–57). London: Oxford University Press.
Punt, N. (1967). *The singer's and actor's throat*. London: Heinemann.
Renfrew, C., Mitchell, J., & Wallace, A (1957). Listening. *Speech, 21,* 34–38.
Riddell, V. (1970). Thyroidectomy: Prevention of recurrent laryngeal nerve palsy. *British Journal of Surgery, 57,* 1–11.
Rippon, T., & Fletcher, P. (1940). *Reassurance and relaxation*. London: Routledge.
Robbins, J., Fisher, H., & Logemann, J. (1982). Acoustic characteristics of voice production after Staffieri's surgical reconstructive procedure. *Journal of Speech and Hearing Disorders, 47,* 77–84.
Robe, E., Brumlik, J., & Moore, P. (1960). A study of spastic dysphonia. *Laryngoscope, 70,* 219–245.
Schaeffer, S. (1983). Neuropathology of spastic dysphonia. *Laryngoscope, 93,* 1183–1204.
Scott, S., & Caird, F. (1983). The response of the apparent receptive speech disorder of Parkinson's disease to speech therapy. *Journal of Neurology, Neurosurgery, and Psychiatry, 47,* 302–304.
Selby, G. (1967). Stereotactic surgery for the relief of Parkinson's disease. *Journal of the Neurological Sciences, 5,* 343–375.
Selley, W. (1977). Dental help for stroke patients. *British Dental Journal, 141,* 409–412.
Sessions, D., Maness, G., & McSwain, B. (1965). Laryngofissure in the treatment of carcinoma of the vocal cord: A report of 40 cases and a review of the literature. *Laryngoscope, 75,* 490–502.
Seth, G., & Guthrie, D. (1935). *Speech in childhood*. London: Oxford University Press.
Shaw, H. (1966). Partial laryngectomy. *Journal of Laryngology and Otology, 80,* 839–850.
Shepperd, H. (1966). Androgenic hoarseness. *Journal of Laryngology and Otology, 80,* 403–405.
Singer, M., & Blom, E. (1980). An endoscopic technique for restoration of voice after laryngectomy. *Annals of Oto-Rhino-Laryngology, 89,* 529–533.
Singer, M., & Blom, E. (1983). Restoration of voice after total laryngectomy. In G. English (Ed.), *Otolaryngology* (Vol. 5, Chap. 37, pp. 1–10). Philadelphia: Lippincott.
Snidecor, J. (1968). *Speech rehabilitation of the laryngectomized*. Springfield, IL: Thomas.
Sonninen, A. (1960). Laryngeal signs and symptoms of goitre. *Folia Phoniatrica, 12,* 41–47.
Sonninen, A., Damsté, R., & Fokkens, J. (1972). On vocal strain. *Folia Phoniatrica, 24,* 321–336.
Sørenson, H. (1982). Laser surgery in benign laryngeal disease. *Acta Oto-Laryngologica, 94,* 537–540.
Staffieri, M. (1980). New surgical approaches for speech rehabilitation after total laryngectomy. In D. Shedd & B. Weinberg (Eds.), *Surgical and prosthetic approaches to speech rehabilitation* (pp. 77–118). Boston: Hall Medical Publications.
Sundberg, J. (1970). Formant structure and articulation of spoken and sung vowels. *Folia Phoniatrica, 22,* 28–48.

Taub, S. (1975). Air bypass prosthesis for vocal rehabilitation of laryngectomees. *Annals of Oto-Rhino-Laryngology, 84*, 45–48.

Toohill, R. (1975). The psychosomatic aspects of children with vocal nodules. *Archives of Otolaryngology, 101*, 591–595.

Tudor, C., & Selley, W. (1974). A palatal training appliance and a visual speech aid for use in hypernasal speech. *British Journal of Disorders of Communication, 9*, 117–122.

Van den Berg, J. (1962). Modern research in experimental phonetrics. *Folia Phoniatrica, 14*, 81–149.

Van den Berg, J. (1964). Some physical aspects of voice production. In D. Brewer (Ed.), *Research potentials in voice physiology* (pp. 63–101). Syracuse: State University of New York, Upstate Medical Center.

Vaughn, C., & Strong, M. (1983). Benign lesions of the larynx. In G. English (Ed.), *Otolaryngology* (Vol. 5, Chap. 33, pp. 1–29). New York: Lippincott.

Von Leden, H., Yanagihara, N., & Werner-Kukuk, E. (1967). Teflon in unilateral vocal cord paralysis. *Archives of Otolaryngology, 85*, 666–674.

Weiss, D. (1950). The pubertal changes of the human voice (mutation). *Folia Phoniatrica, 2*, 127–158.

Weiss, D. (1960). Therapy of cluttering. *Folia Phoniatrica, 12*, 216–213.

Weiss, D. (1964). *Cluttering*. Englewood Cliffs, NJ: Prentice-Hall.

Weiss, D., & Beebe, H. (1951). *The chewing approach in speech and voice therapy*. New York: Karger.

Wilder, C. (1983). Chest wall preparation for phonation in female speakers. In D. Bliss & J. Abbs (Eds.), *Vocal fold physiology* (pp. 109–123). San Diego: College Hill Press.

Wilson, D. (1962). Voice reeducation of children with vocal nodules. *Laryngoscope, 72*, 45–53.

Wilson, D. (1979). *Voice problems of children*. Baltimore: Williams & Wilkins.

Wolfe, V., Garvin, J., Bacon, M., & Waldrop, W. (1975). Speech changes in Parkinson's disease during treatment with L-dopa. *Journal of Communication Disorders, 8*, 271–279.

Wyke, B. (1969). Deus ex machina vocis: An analysis of laryngeal reflexes in speech. *British Journal of Disorders of Communication, 4*, 3–25.

Wyke, B. (1974). Laryngeal muscular control systems in singing: A review of current concepts. *Folia Phoniatrica, 26*, 249–264.

Wynter, H., & Martin, S. (1981). The classification of deviant voice quality through auditory memory. *British Journal of Disorders of Communication, 16*, 204–210.

Wynn-Williams, D. (1958). Congenital supra bulbar paresis. *Speech Pathology and Therapy, 1*, 18–24.

Zilstorff, K. (1968). Vocal disabilities of singers. *Proceedings of the Royal Society of Medicine, 61*, 1147–1150.

**Margaret Greene** is a Fellow of the College of Speech Therapists in London. She has been Head of Department at Stoke Mandeville Hospital in Aylesbury, followed by a similar post at St. Bartholomew's Hospital in London. She was Director of Studies at the Central School of Speech and Drama for the speech pathologists' training course. She remains, after retirement, consultant speech therapist to the Department of Medical Electronics at St. Bartholomew's, with special interests in respiratory patterns and electronic speech aids. She is the founder and vice-president of the Association for All Speech Impaired Children (AFASIC). She has regularly presented papers at national conferences and contributed articles and chapters to many major publications. She is best known for *The Voice and Its Disorders*. Her considerable writing output reflects a knowledge of international developments in speech pathology as well as experience gained during lecture tours in Australia, New Zealand, India, and South Africa as a guest of the various speech and hearing associations.

**DATE DUE**

| OC 7 '00 | | | |
|---|---|---|---|
| | | | |
| | | | |
| | | | |
| | | | |
| | | | |
| | | | |
| | | | |
| | | | |
| | | | |
| | | | |

RF 510 .G73 1986

57657

Greene, Margaret C.L.
Disorders of voice.

HIEBERT LIBRARY
Fresno Pacific College - M. B. Seminary
Fresno, Calif. 93702